A Jesus Girl's Guide to Healing Your Food and Weight Struggles

By Amy Suliano Cox

Copyright © 2017 by Amy Suliano Cox

All rights reserved. This book or any portion thereof may not be reproduced or used in any manner whatsoever without the express written permission of the publisher.

ISBN-13: 978-1546465577
ISBN-10: 154646557X

Contents

Introduction 1

My Story 9

Chapter 1: What Is Your Why? 19

Chapter 2: What Do You Believe About Yourself? 27

Chapter 3: Intentional Thoughts = Desired Goals 37

Chapter 4: Learning to Listen to Your Body 47

Chapter 5: How to Feel Your Feelings and Stop Eating Them 57

Chapter 6: Movement as Praise 67

Chapter 7: Applying God's Word 77

Chapter 8: A Lens of Gratitude 89

Chapter 9: Be Still and Know 97

Chapter 10: Mercy and Grace 105

Chapter 11: My Prayer for You 113

Introduction

Hello, sweet sister. I'm guessing you've picked up this book because you are tired: tired of this battle with your weight, tired of feeling out of control around food, tired of feeling broken and lost, tired of food playing such a huge role in your life. I understand. I know you worry sometimes if anything is going to work for you long-term. I know you've tried it all: the diets, the tricks, the cleanses, and the exercise plans. You've deprived yourself, white-knuckled it. You've tried things that you're ashamed to even admit, yet none of them have worked long-term. You've seen progress on some levels, yet your weight still shows the world that you are struggling, that something isn't quite right. You are still battling against yourself. You fear the struggle means that you are incapable, and you have doubts about your ability to have lasting change. You worry that you will always struggle no matter what, so you give up on some level. You feel like each failure is just another reminder of how you will never get it right, how freedom from your weight and eating struggles is just not possible for you, and how no one else could ever understand what being you is like. You flounder between acceptance and wanting more.

I hear you, and I feel you. I also know that beneath those worries and fears lies a little bit of hope that an answer exists that you haven't uncovered yet. Your heart is good, and you want to change—to care for yourself. You want the battle to end. You *know* in your heart of hearts that you are missing out on something by continuing to be distracted by this struggle. You've battled at times with yourself and with God, trying to understand what all of this means and what all of this is for. You know He has a plan for you. You know He doesn't allow struggle into your life without a purpose, but you still don't know what that purpose is, and you've grown tired. The battle seems long at times. The cross feels heavy. The thorn stings. You sometimes wish to wake up and find this burden taken from you: the weight, the struggle, and the pain. You wish that you could look at food as just that, food. Sometimes, you do. Sometimes, food is enjoyable without the struggle. You like fueling yourself with healthy stuff. You like the way your body feels when everything is clicking. You experience that level of deciding what is best for you from a loving and healthy place.

Unfortunately, you also have disconnected times that seem to come out of nowhere. You check out. Your brain seems like it can only focus on food, and nothing else seems to satisfy that desire. You find yourself standing in front of the pantry trying this and eating that. You find yourself at the bottom of a bag of chips, but you still feel empty, or you eat until the familiar feeling of fullness sets in. You don't know why, but the physical feeling of discomfort feels comfortable to you. It's a feeling you know and understand. You ask yourself, "Does it really matter if I overeat? Who cares if I use food to comfort or distract myself? Who am I really hurting anyway?"

You know the truth that deep down, you are hurting yourself. You know deep down that it *does* matter, but how do you get past those doubts in the moment? How do you trust that the bigger picture is important enough for you to face your fears? How do you trust God to make good out of this struggle? Do you believe in His ability to help you conquer this internal battle and to create purpose out of it all?

Terry came to me with this problem. She felt like she

was "supposed" to lose weight, but she was tired of trying. She had experienced some success in the past with losing weight. She had tried Weight Watchers, Nutrisystem, low-carb diets, and gluten-free diets. She had lost different amounts of weight with each diet plan, but she would eventually gain it all back. She felt destined to struggle with her weight and food forever. She came to me to start exercising consistently but wasn't quite ready to address the food struggle. She was almost resigned to the fact that she just loved to eat food, and she didn't see a problem with it.

As we dug deeper and worked on why she overate, the story of the role food played in her life unfolded a bit more. Food was her comfort. Food was the one thing she could depend on and control in her life. When her emotions and the environment around her seemed out of her control, food was her friend. She knew what to expect from food, and she knew it would give her a chance to forget whatever she was going through, even if just for a little while. She wondered if overeating really mattered. Her health was fine. Yes, she had excess weight on her body, but she just wasn't sure losing the weight mattered to her anymore. She wasn't sure that she wanted to stop overeating, so that's where her work began.

This may be the starting point for you too. You may need to ask yourself if getting control of your weight matters enough to you. Are you open to healing the parts of yourself that still struggle with food and your weight? Are you open to learning how to do this differently? Are you willing to connect with what you really want for yourself and with the purpose for which God has created you? You know He cares about you, right? He cares that you hurt. He cares that you struggle. He wants you to turn to Him, lean on Him, and trust in Him, not food. He cares so much that He has equipped you with everything you need for this journey. He has gone ahead of you and paved your way. He knows every stumbling block, every victory, and every failure you will encounter. He will use *every* one of those things for your benefit. He will help you to see that through Him all things are possible, that nothing is off limits from His power and ability, that you are His, that you matter, and that you are important! Everything going on in your life—every struggle, every tear, every laugh, every moment—is everything to Him. He created you for a purpose—a mighty purpose,—and He's asking you to show up, or react, in a different way. You have accepted Jesus as your Savior. You have turned away from your past hurts and sins and given them all over to Him. The Holy Spirit *lives* in you. He wants you to listen to the still, small voice inside yourself that tells you to believe in Him. He wants you to not only connect to His voice, but to move forward from that place of love. He is waiting to help you. He wants to reveal Himself to you in every situation.

Let's go back to Terry and her problem. She struggled at first with why God would care about this part of her life. "Doesn't He have bigger things to worry about?" she would ask. "I've failed at this so many times. He has to have given up on me at this point too." Because she had in some ways given up on herself, she truly believed He had too.

Compartmentalizing this area in her life was "easier" than going to Him with it. Instead, she tried to fix it all on her own, but sometimes her fears of failure were so overwhelming, she would be too paralyzed to do anything. She didn't know how to take any different action.

Are your fears stopping you as well? Are you replaying all the times in your life that you've started a new plan, made a new promise to yourself, or committed yourself to trying again? Are you remembering the failures and the times that you thought you had it all figured out and then stumbled? Have you lost yourself or your way? I know these stumbles can seem so hard from which to recover. Sometimes, life throws unexpected things at you: things that you aren't prepared for and didn't even see coming. You think you have it all figured out, and then the script changes—life changes. You don't know how to recover or how to move on. You've learned not to beat yourself up too badly when things happen and circumstances are outside of your control. You've started looking at these situations as opportunities to learn and grow. The black-and-white thinking has turned a little grayer. Things aren't quite as clear-cut as you used to think. While this is empowering, it's also confusing at times, and the confusion can become the new stumbling block. You don't know how to proceed in these moments, so you just don't move at all. Fear creeps back in, and you think it means that something is wrong or missing.

I'm here to tell you that nothing is wrong. Nothing is missing. You are *exactly* who you are meant to be at this very moment in time. God can and *will* use every detail of this very moment to move you forward and to make your path clear. All you have to do is ask, get still, and become aware. Open your heart to the guidance of His spirit. Understand that your mind is within your control (as opposed to being a helpless victim of your thoughts) and that your body is your friend. Remember that when you connect your mind, body, and spirit fully with God's truth, you are in alignment with Him; and when you feel lost, uncertain, fearful, and confused, this place of alignment with God's love and promises is where you need to come back to. He has equipped you with everything you need. You have the Holy Spirit living inside you; you just have to listen and connect with Him. This is the place of healing.

I'm here to help you, to guide you along the way, to remind you of the Light when the darkness sets in, to remind you that God has everything under control and has an amazing plan for you, to be your cheerleader and confidant, to ask you questions that help you uncover the next layer, and to celebrate with you when you discover God's enabling power. You know that you are different and that what works for someone else may not work for you. You are ready to move past the level of needing to fit into someone else's box. Now is the time to write your own journey. Now is the time to define what healthy means for you and to be okay with redefining what that is when the seasons in your life change. The struggle to this point has been trying to fit into the "one size fits all" mentality and feeling like a failure when you can't fit, but you're ready. You know a different way has to exist.

Reaching this level of understanding is what finally enabled Terry to step forward. She was able to see that she was made to connect with God and that when she addressed all areas of herself—mind, body, and spirit—in this fashion, she could use every opportunity to learn, grow, and trust God and herself. From this place of close communion, she was able to begin the work of healing her struggles.

So trust and believe in your next step. Trust in your ability to figure out what works for you and believe that you are capable. Trust that this new way will work for you—that you can adopt this method to fit the uniqueness of you. The only thing that has been missing between you and your relationship with yourself is the understanding and awareness of how all of this is connected—how your mind, body, and spirit can work together for your greatest good. When you make this connection and intentionally align these pieces of yourself with God's truth, love, and promises, everything comes together. When one of these elements is a little off, you have an opportunity to learn. It's not a failure. You are capable of turning and following God's guidance in your heart.

Let's take these steps together: learn the tools that will help you along your path; understand the trustworthiness of the internal guidance of the Holy Spirit; connect to God's truth, love, and promises for your life; and know that you serve a great purpose on this earth. You are not here by accident. No mistakes were made leading up to this very day. God has picked you specifically for a purpose. No coincidences exist in life, and you are reading this book for a reason! Trust in Him and this divine moment before you. Commit your heart to Him and move forward knowing that your steps will be clear, that you will know exactly what to do, and that all of the dreams and desires placed within you will be achieved as you walk daily with Him (Pr. 37:4).

My Story

I can vividly remember standing in front of the pantry unwrapping the next Little Debbie snack before I had even finished the first one. I was not a picky Little Debbie girl either. I liked them all: Swiss Rolls, Nutty Bars, Oatmeal Pies, Fudge Rounds. If the name Little Debbie was on it, I ate it. I seemed to have a big, giant hole within me that needed filling, and food became my filler of choice. My preteen years were the beginning of my trying to figure out how I fit into the world. Unfortunately, my increasing weight became part of how I defined myself. The world made clear to me that my weight was an issue and that "big-boned" was not a compliment. The little comments here and there that I either overhead or were said directly to me about being fat stung. For a young girl who already had a high level of confusion in her life, reconciling who I was in the world became even more difficult because I viewed myself as a failure because of my weight. The result? I would eat.

Looking back on the facts of my life and seeing how I created my story around them is interesting. I was the child of divorced parents and was raised Catholic. In hindsight, those details really are not that big of a deal, but the story I created around these circumstances stayed with me through adulthood. I remember always identifying myself as the product of a divorce and trying to explain to my friends how that worked, having half siblings, stepparents, and separate families. I felt stuck between two worlds and two loyalties. As a child, I made the divorce mean a lot about who I was in the world and how different I was from my friends. Most of their parents were still married, and they lived with their siblings. They did not quite understand the dynamics of divorce, so I got really good at compartmentalizing all of those areas of my life.

Being raised Catholic played a very big part in my story as well. I went to a Catholic school as a young child and learned my basics about Jesus and Christianity from there. My "divorce story" was not helped since the Church was very vocal on its stance regarding divorce, and even as a young child, I picked up on the fact that it was regarded as wrong. What I took away from my early teachings of faith was a deep level of guilt and never feeling quite up to par. My first connection with Christ was the reminder of His death on the cross, represented in a crucifix hung vividly for young eyes to ponder above the altar at Mass. My sense of God at this point was that of a disappointed dad. I knew He loved me, but I was constantly reminded of how I was not living up to His standards. I did not quite get the understanding that Jesus had wiped away all of my sin and shame and that I did not have to earn His approval. I am not sure if my young mind just could not comprehend the truth, or if it was never taught to me in that way.

My desire to please was born. The life of an emotional eating perfectionist had begun. I wanted so desperately to please my parents, my family, and God. I think I used food because I did not know how else to handle my emotions as a child. Food became the easy way to give myself comfort and to help me feel some semblance of control in my life. In hindsight, I am not surprised I had weight and food issues. I had placed the weight of the world on my shoulders by thinking that I was responsible for everyone around me, and then I felt guilty when I messed up and was not perfect. When I added the feeling of being a total failure to God, I had a distorted understanding of where my worth came from. I had set myself up for failure from the start in believing that I had to have it all together to please or gain acceptance from God and those around me. To be honest, this is the world's message, not God's. God says, "Believe in the Lord Jesus Christ, and you will be saved" (Acts 16:31; Rom. 10:9).

I was your typical, overachieving, smart girl throughout high school and college. I had my moments of wayward paths and bad decision-making, but my guilty conscious would eventually lead me back to perfectionism, a standard I would always fall short of but that kept me striving to be better. When I would fail or falter, I would eat. I guess in some ways I am grateful that my desires to better myself were so strong, because they did give me opportunities to grow and learn. I just wish that young girl had known that she did not have to be perfect for love and acceptance. Those were already hers for the taking. God was waiting patiently for her to see that.

In a similar way, I am extremely grateful that I had a sense of faith and God from a very early age even though I used this faith on an "as needed" basis for most of my life. When things were bad, I would cry out to God, but I never quite understood that I could depend on Him for everything and at all times. The thought never crossed my mind that He wanted to help me with the things that caused my emotional eating. I just chalked my desire to eat up to an imperfection—one more way I was not hitting the mark.

Don't get me wrong. I knew that God was my answer. I just thought I had to be perfect before I could turn to Him. The faulty belief that I had compartmentalized as a child told me that if I just tried harder, if I just got my act together, if I just fixed myself, then I could come to Him without being a hypocrite. I could claim His work over my life. I would be good enough.

My weight struggles continued into my junior year of college at the University of Mississippi where I experienced my first real taste of weight loss. Fen-phen and the low-fat diet craze were really popular at the time, and the combination of diet and drug seemed to be the perfect experience. I had fen-phen to suppress my appetite so that I did not have to deal with hunger cravings, and I had fat-free Pop-Tarts, Cool Whip, and Gummy Savers to fulfill my childhood love of sugar.

I lost weight, and I lost weight fast! I am not going to lie—it felt pretty awesome—until the world found out that fen-phen was bad for your heart, and fat-free did not mean calorie-free or healthy. What's the saying? "If it sounds too good to be true, it probably is." I also started working out (and enjoying it) for the first time in my life. After years of trying to skip every PE class and embarrassing myself with my lack of athletic talent in childhood sports, I found that I actually enjoyed going to the gym and exercising. I was, of course, still hiding out in the deserted women's-only section of my college-town gym, but baby steps were being made!

Unfortunately, my appetite returned in full force without fen-phen, and the weight crept back on. This continued for the next ten years, which I lovingly refer to as my yo-yo dieting years. See, before that I had just been overweight. No yo-yoing was involved because I had never really tried the whole losing weight thing (unless you include taking laxatives for two days at fourteen years old and then being so scared that I was going to die that I never tried it again). I spent the next ten years trying *all* of the different diets. I would have some success, but eventually put the weight (plus some) back on. Eventually, in my early 30s, I was just done. I was so tired of being overweight and of being *that* girl who just could not get the diet and exercise thing figured out. I was exhausted with the weight (physically and mentally) that this struggle produced.

I started Weight Watchers again and knew that I needed to get the exercise part down too. I started going to the gym and taking some classes, but I needed more guidance than that. I was surfing the Weight Watchers online boards when I came across an "ask the trainer" post. It was for an online personal trainer (Corinne with Phit-N-Phat), and I started stalking her website and blog. I was more of a looker, but I put in my application to her program and online community, and I literally felt like I had won the golden ticket when I got accepted. This started my journey of learning how to exercise and make it a part of my daily life. This was my first experience with having a support system around me that understood my struggles and was there to support me on my journey. My weight loss continued, and I truly felt like I was on the right track. Health and fitness were becoming my passions.

At this same time, I was also struggling with what my true purpose in life was. I was stuck in a job that provided very little fulfillment. Yes, I was using my degree. Yes, I was making good money. Yes, I was skilled and good at what I was doing, but I still had this ache in my heart for more to my life than this. This was the first time I was really able to hear that yearning in my heart for more, and I truly believe that it was because I was finally dealing with the surface weight issue. Without realizing it at the time, I was losing that first layer of mental weight that had been holding me back from stepping further into who God had created me to be. Up until that point, I had followed the life plan. I had graduated from college, started a career, and gotten married, but my weight had been holding me back from feeling like I was worthy of pursuing anything outside the "norm."

I finally bit the bullet, quit my job, and got certified as a personal trainer. Not only did becoming a personal trainer allow me a new career opportunity, but it was also a chance to help other women who struggled with the same issues as me, and my servant's heart loved this idea. Subconsciously, I also thought being a trainer would be a great accountability tool for keeping the weight off. Even though I had finally had success at losing weight, I still did not trust myself to keep it off.

My subconscious was partially right because my struggles with emotional eating were far from over. Losing more than eighty pounds and building a business helping other women lose weight had provided a lot of knowledge into *how* to lose weight, but it had not addressed *why* food continued to be a battle. My habit was still to turn to food for comfort, control, and distraction, so my desire for self-improvement continued. I struggled a lot during this season, trying to understand where God fit into all this and why the burden of emotional eating was so hard for me to figure out. Many times I felt that having to bear such a public "cross" was unfair, that I could never hide my internal struggling, and that I was being judged every time I stepped in front of a client or told someone I was a personal trainer.

I eventually started listening to a podcast called *The Life Coach School* and was introduced to how our brains are conditioned to work as well as how our thoughts are connected to the results we have in our lives. I knew that not only was this insight into the next step in my own personal development, but it would also help my clients bridge the gap between understanding the diet and exercise portion of weight loss and the mind work that was essential for the weight loss journey to be life-changing and lifelong. The podcast truly was a missing piece to the puzzle that allowed me to move forward in a way that was empowering and divinely guided.

You see, all of this work was the starting place for me to finally make the mind, body, spirit connection. I was beginning to understand how the box into which I kept trying to fit God was as ridiculous as thinking fen-phen and a low-fat diet would have no side effects. A real understanding of how everything fit together finally happened: that one could not function fully without the other. Healing was available when my mind, body, and spirt were in alignment with Him. The struggles of my life came full circle when I addressed my mindset, honored my body, and connected with my Source.

Looking back on my years of struggle, God was always present and woven into each of these areas of my life. I was just too busy trying to fix everything on my own to see His presence. I was not aware that He had already provided me with all of the knowledge I needed to believe Him for what He promised: to get me through *any* situation in life. I was still that young Catholic girl thinking that I had to fix all these problems myself before I could be worthy enough to stand before Him with my life.

Thankfully, He has continued to work on my heart to let Him in, to give Him the broken pieces of my life, and to stop trying to put the puzzle together without His help. He is capable of making a much more beautiful picture of it all if I just let Him, and He has. He has shown me how to love myself fully, to give myself grace when needed, to have gratitude in every situation, to honor this gift of life He has given me, and to serve with a heart that understands. He has made the most beautiful message out of the mess of a young Jesus girl's heart.

~Your life is your story. Write well, edit often.

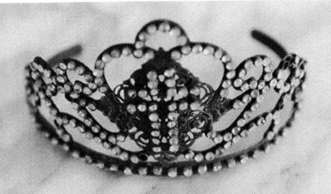

and do not be conformed to this world but be transformed by the renewing of your mind so that you may prove what the will of God is that which is good acceptable and perfect

romans 12:12

Chapter 1: What Is Your Why?

Have you ever taken the time to get really clear on why you want to lose weight? Why you want to stop emotionally eating? What is it that you think will come from dropping the weight and having a healthy relationship with food? Getting clear on why we want this change in our lives is so instrumental in understanding what we make this weight/food struggle mean about us. Figuring out the underlying story that we tell ourselves about why losing weight and getting healthy is so important is key in beginning to win the battle.

For most of us, the answer to why seems pretty straightforward on the surface: to look better, to feel better, to be healthier, to be able to wear cute clothes, etc. These appear to be good enough reasons, right? The bigger question, though, is why do you want to focus on feeling better, being healthier, and looking better? There is more to the story then these simple answers, and usually the answer is a lot deeper than you would have ever considered.

Wanting to lose weight, feel healthy, or end the cycle of emotional eating is not wrong, but chances are you have wanted these things for a while now, yet you have not been able to achieve them long-term. Understanding your true *why* is instrumental in understanding your mind-set when setting these health and weight-loss goals for yourself. Whatever thoughts, worries, fears, and hopes are driving your goals are also going to directly affect the actions you take and, ultimately, the results you get.

One of the ways I help my clients determine why they have set the goals that they have is to walk them through an exercise called the "The 5 *Whys*." This technique is used throughout the personal development world, but strangely enough, it started in the manufacturing industry to help identify the root cause of production problems. This strategy asks five repetitive *whys* in a question-and-answer method. You start by making your first *why* whatever your primary goal is: Why do I want to be healthy and lose weight? Why do I want to exercise? Why do I want to stop emotionally eating? Then, the answer to that question becomes the next question to be answered and so forth. Here's one that I filled out for myself several years ago:

- Why do I want to be healthy? Because I want to take care of myself and live a long, healthy life.
- Why do I want to take care of myself and live a long, healthy life? Because I want to set a good example for those around me that I love.
- Why do I want to set a good example for those around me that I love? Because I want them to take care of themselves and be around for a long time.
- Why do I want them to take care of themselves and be around for a long time? Because I do not want to lose them.
- Why do I not want to lose them? Because I do not want to be alone.

The underlying why is not quite as clear-cut as it would seem, right? Our desires and goals are usually so much more than just being able to wear a certain size pair of jeans or weigh a certain amount on the scale. Ultimately, that mind-set—my fear of being alone—did not help me to feel motivated in the hard times. In fact, it would paralyze me, and the cycle of emotional eating would continue because I wanted so badly not to feel that fear and worry. Does this mean that now I do not worry about losing my loved ones or being alone? Not exactly. But it did give me the framework for understanding the story I was creating around what being healthy meant for me and, ultimately, what I was afraid of. One thing I have learned for myself is that fear is not the best emotion for me to make decisions from or to be motivated from. I have learned to switch the focus of my "why" to an empowering feeling that allows me to make decisions from a place of peace, confidence, and joy.

One of the ways to change your focus is to figure out how you want to feel when you have reached your goals. What do you envision this process will bring you? A feeling of confidence, peace, or joy? What will be different about you? What will be the same? Take a few minutes and visualize yourself one year from now. Are you at your natural weight? What are you wearing? How do you feel around your favorite foods? What do you think about yourself after reaching your goals? List two to four words that would describe who you are at that moment. How do these words resonate with you? Is there one that speaks to you on a different level more than the others do?

Pick one word to be your guiding word on this journey. What one word would best describe how you would like to feel after finishing this book and making these steps a part of your daily life? This word will be your touchstone as you make these life changes. This word can help bring you back to your dream of what is possible for yourself. This word can be the way you start to live today, right now, in this very moment.

My client, Pam, is a great example of how this works.

She was ready to make a lasting change and wanted to do it differently than before. She knew that her ability to be successful would need to come from a different focus and a different source. She chose the word "peace" for her journey. She was ready to stop battling herself, to end the suffering her weight struggles created, and to create a healthy view of herself. She identified the Bible verses Galatians 5:22–23, "But the fruit of the Spirit is love, joy, peace, forbearance, kindness, goodness, faithfulness, gentleness, and self-control," as verses that spoke to who she wanted to be as a result of her goals. She used these verses and her guiding word of peace to focus on the "why" of what was important to her: why she was choosing to love herself in a different way, why she believed that her ability to do things differently this time would work, and why she wanted to change. She found that this word helped her to stay focused on her goals because her *why* was true peace for herself.

The beautiful thing about doing the healing around your *why* is understanding where your deepest desires come from—clarity. Making goals and moving toward a certain focus is wonderful, but clarity on the matter brings about a different level of awareness and how you can show up differently when you can get clear on your motivation. I am not promoting some "woo-woo" experience. What we focus on grows, so if your focus is on a place of love and peace, you will experience love and peace for yourself. If your focus is on a place of fear or unworthiness, you will experience that instead.

Write your word down as a reminder. Get a pretty bracelet with the word on it, or paint a rock with your word to remind you of why this journey is so important to you. Where can you start experiencing this feeling in your life right now?

Make this your daily mantra—your feeling on which to meditate. Is there a Bible verse that speaks to this desired feeling? Write it out on a bookmark to use. Come back to this verse each and every day and set your intentions for the day to that desired feeling. When you are choosing how to eat that day, think of your word. When you are tired and do not feel like exercising, go back to your verse. Remind yourself of the promise God has made, and then ask yourself what you should do differently according to that verse. The closer you can come to making your decisions from this place of emotion, the closer you will be to your goals.

Now, you need to do a little goal setting. What are your ultimate goals for your mind, body, and spirit? To define what healthy looks like to you, you need to start with what your expectations are. If all of your dreams were to come true today, how would your mind be? How would your body and spirit be? Would you be focusing on things that are negative and frustrate you? Would you be eating things that make your body feel a certain way? Would you be filling your mind with God's Word? What practices would you have in place to align yourself in a healthy manner?

One of the struggles we have today is trying to live up to what the world defines as healthy. We look at what the world tells us we should do to be healthy, what size we should be, and what is required from us to be worthy, acceptable, and enough. God gives us these definitions clearly. He guides us in honoring our bodies as God's temple, in renewing our minds on a daily basis, and in using the power of the Holy Spirit in our lives. Imagine defining healthy for yourself in God's terms. What has He put on your heart to work on? How does He want you to take care of yourself? How can you look to His internal guidance to determine what healthy means for you? How can you align what you want for yourself with what will bring you closer to whom God created you to be?

I worked with my client, Tina, to identify her new "healthy her" mission statement. She had tried to fit into the mold that society had told her to for many years and was tired of missing that mark. She was willing to dig a little deeper and trust in her ability to decide what she wanted her healthy life to look like. She decided to make a new mission statement for her life. Here is what she discovered she wanted most: "Healthy for me is when my mind, body, and spirit are aligned. I am living intentionally, authentically, and joyfully. There is a balance in my life of love, laughter, growing, learning, sweating, nourishing foods, and Jesus. A healthy mind for me is always growing and learning, considering other perspectives, being open to change, but owning who I am and what I choose to think without defensiveness or judgement. Health for my body looks like nourishment, love, care, moving, a healthy relationship with my temple, and ownership of how I'm designed. Healthy for my spirit is connection, personal, quiet, stillness, intuitiveness, holy, peace."

- What does healthy look like for you? Get clear on how you want to define healthy for you.
- What is your *why*? Identify what the underlying reason is for why you want to lose weight.
- What guiding word will be your touch stone along this journey? Write your word down, come back to it daily, and be intentional with your decision-making around this desired word.

~Know your why. This is the driving force behind everything.

Chapter 2: What Do You Believe About Yourself?

Have you ever started a diet on a Monday thinking, *This time it will be different*, only to fear failure from the start? Have you stood on the scale feeling defeated by the number glaring back at you? Have your thoughts ever gone to, *I am such a failure. Once again, I've fallen off the wagon, and here I stand on this piece of metal with proof of how I don't quite measure up. I will never be able to change. Why can't I just get this right? What is wrong with me?* Has the voice in your head ever sounded like this?

- *I am broken.*
- *I am lazy.*
- *I am lost.*
- *I am tired.*
- *I am stupid.*
- *I am fat.*
- *I am a failure.*
- *I am a mess.*
- *I am incapable.*
- *I am always going to be fat.*
- *Why even try?*

I have some very important questions for you, my friend. What do you believe about yourself? What do you say to yourself in the privacy of your own mind? Does a dialogue of self-defeat play in your head like a broken record? Even when you find that new diet plan, are you intrigued, yet doubtful? Does the interest in a new plan inspire you to change in the beginning but get drowned out by your fears of failure? Do you often start a new plan already unsure of your ability to succeed? Do you wonder why you get a taste of success and then sabotage your efforts? Do you feel stuck wondering, *Why can't I do this? Why do I always self-destruct? What is wrong with me?*

The only thing wrong, my friend, is that you keep looking outside of yourself for the answer. You think a diet or exercise routine will provide the answer and freedom you are desperately seeking. You are conditioned to believe these random *I am* thoughts without realizing that thinking this way is what makes you feel defeated and broken. You have bought into the message that you are not enough, not worthy, and not loved. You do not realize that the only thing stopping you from changing is the lies you keep telling yourself, the story that you have created about who you are, and that internal bully that keeps "reminding" you of all the reasons why you cannot succeed.

Can you agree today to shut off the internal bully? Can you move forward in this journey. Are you willing to be kind to yourself no matter what? Will you stay open to challenging every thought that comes into your mind and speaking to yourself in a way that empowers you through God's truth?

Please, take comfort in the fact that God designed you in all of your perfectly imperfect uniqueness (Psalms 139:13–16). He is also the one who knew you would struggle, knew you would fail, and wanted you to have His promise of redemption from the beginning. It is right there for you, waiting for you to believe it. He has declared hope, prosperity, freedom, and redemption over your life. "'For I know the plans I have for you,' says the Lord, 'plans to prosper you and not to harm you, plans to give you a hope and a future'" (Jer. 29:11). He does not say, "I have plans for you only when you get your act together." He does not say He will prosper you when you finally figure out how to stop distracting yourself with food. He says He has these plans for you in spite of all of your quirks, hang-ups, and struggles. He knows your human self is going to struggle, but He wants you to understand that the plans He has for you include all of those struggles, that He has redeemed you already, and that you just have to believe His promises to you.

To begin believing, you have to be willing to shut off the lies you are telling yourself, the ones that the enemy (Satan) uses to distract you from the truth, the ones that tell you that God's promises are not really for you. They are for others, those who have life all figured out. Please, promise to stop allowing these lies to pull you away from Him. Please, stay open to learning a new way to talk to yourself, a new way to define who you *really* are. When you allow your focus to be on these distractions, you look to comfort yourself outside of God. You look to food to lean on instead of God. You falsely believe that your feelings are so wrong you cannot take them to Him and that He is too busy to care about this part of your life.

He says otherwise. He tells us that He cares about everything going on with us—all of it—including the fight you just had with your husband and the frustration over what your mom just said to you. He even cares about the judgement you feel at not being able to lose weight. He wants you to bring these problems to Him (I Peter. 5:7), to lean on Him, to allow these feelings to be processed, and to remember what He has already declared regarding you: hope and prosperity.

While He does not cause the difficulties in our lives, He does allow them as an opportunity to develop our character and our relationship with Him (Rom. 8:28), so how do you change the negative thoughts you have about yourself? First, you have to identify them. You cannot change what you are unwilling to acknowledge. You cannot bring light to a situation that you are trying to keep in the dark. Draw back the curtains and shine a spotlight on your thoughts. Be honest and real with yourself and with Him. He already knows what you think about yourself, but do *you* know what you really think? Are you fully conscious of how you judge yourself and criticize your every move? You cannot believe His truth for you if it differs from what you say about yourself. If you want real change, you have to grab hold of His truth.

Grab a pen and some paper and write down everything you think of when you read these next few questions. No judgement and no editing, just let the thoughts flow.

- Do you believe you can lose weight once and for all?
- Why do you think you struggle with your weight and food?
- What comes to your mind when I say, "You are worthy"?
- What do you think when I say, "You are capable"?
- What are your thoughts about the role food plays in your life?
- What do you say to yourself when you stand on the scale?
- What do you say to yourself when you wear shorts?
- What do you say to yourself when you stand naked?
- What words come to your mind when you are in a

bathing suit?
- What do you believe about your abilities to be in a room full of your favorite foods by yourself when you are sad, mad, angry, and/or fearful?
- Do you believe in God's ability to heal your weight and food struggles?

I want you to take the time to write all of this out (including whatever else comes up for you with the thought of trying a new approach), and I want you to burn it. Fire to paper—destroy it! Make a ceremony out of it. You can have a bonfire in your backyard or light a candle in the favorite space of your home. I want you to speak out loud that you are done with this way of thinking, that you are ready to believe God for the promises He has for you, and that you will no longer allow the past to hold you back or define what you are capable of doing moving forward. (I would love for you to share this declaration with me. Take a picture of you lighting a fire to what is holding you back and email it to me or tag me on Facebook #iamajesusgirl.)

You are free now. You are free from the lies. You no longer have to hang your head in defeat or think negative things about yourself. You are a child of God. God values you so much that He sent His Son to make a way for you, to provide an opportunity for you to have a personal relationship with Him; and as a daughter of the King, you are able to fully embrace His identity for you (Rom. 8:1-15)! Do you feel the freedom? Can you feel the space you just created for yourself?

Limiting thoughts and feelings no longer have to be a part of your story. You can now move forward with new beliefs in a new direction. This does not have to be some hocus pocus, positive thinking act. You now get to choose to fill your mind with God's truth. This is your opportunity to replace your false beliefs with the truth. As my teacher Brooke Castillo says, "A belief is only a thought you choose to think over and over again." The negative thoughts you had about yourself were only easy to believe because you had them on repeat in your mind.

This is an opportunity to start anew with a clean slate. You get to choose what you will believe about yourself going forward. I am not going to lie to you and say those negative thoughts will never come back up, but stay open to what you will learn in the next chapters as to how to replace those thoughts. You will learn how to consciously choose what you want to think and believe. You now have a fresh start to begin a new process for yourself, to believe God for what He says about you, and to claim the inheritance that is rightly yours. You can adopt a brand-new dialogue that sounds like this:

- I am His (Galatians 3:26).
- I am a new creation (2 Corinthians 5:17).
- I am loved (John 3:16).
- I am fearfully and wonderfully made (Psalm 139:14).
- I am clothed with strength and dignity (Proverbs 31:25).
- I have the power that raised Jesus from the dead living within me (Romans 8:11).
- I am limitless (Philippians 4:13).
- I was created to shine (Matthew 5:16).
- I serve a powerful purpose (Ephesians 2:10).
- I am joy (John 15:11).
- I have self-control (2 Timothy 1:7).
- I am kind (Galatians 5:22).

- He designed me uniquely (Jeremiah 1:4-5).
- I am strong (Isaiah 40:29).
- I am courageous (Joshua 1:9).
- I am worthy (Romans 5:8).

This is your Spirit-given power, my friend. God has given you the ability to think and to choose. You have all of the power you need to change your thinking.

Do you remember Pam? She chose peace as her new focus, her guiding word. She finally believed that peace with her body and relationship with food were possible, and that allowed her to seek true change. Her focus played into every decision she made about herself. When she planned her food out for the week, she planned from a place of peace. When she decided how to exercise each day, she decided with peace in mind. When she weighed herself each week, she aligned with peace first. When she spoke about her lifestyle changes, she spoke from a place of peace. Were there times that required her to refocus? Yes. Did opportunities for struggles present themselves, just like in the past? Absolutely. But her desire for peace continued to motivate her, and she was willing to learn and grow to achieve that peace.

The reason weight loss feels so difficult to you right now is because you have spent years focusing on all the reasons why you cannot do this, why you are a failure, and why food controls you. You think the answer comes from another diet or exercise program. You keep looking outside of yourself instead of receiving the truth of what God says about you and what God is capable of doing through you. You do not need food to play the role of God for you. Food is just a distraction from His truth and His power.

For this new journey to be a success, you must believe

it is possible. Now is the time to think new thoughts about yourself: thoughts that empower you, thoughts that inspire you to be everything that you were created to be, and thoughts that align with God's truth. Your focus is important. The goals you set for yourself in the previous chapter require conscious choice. They are not an attempt to gloss over the reality of your world, but rather, they are there to set your direction to move forward. What you choose to believe and think directly impacts not only your actions but also the results you will experience on your journey. Directing your mind to what is true and holy is choosing to align yourself with God and the gifts He has given you. You have all of the power you need right now to achieve your goals—you just have to believe it.

- With what thoughts are you going to fill your mind today?
- Set your goals every single day and come back to them throughout the day.
- Remind yourself of who God says you are and challenge any thought that is not in alignment with His truth.

~You are what you believe yourself to be.
-Paulo Coelho

Chapter 3: Intentional Thoughts = Desired Goals

"I'm so hungry and frustrated. Why does my mind do this? What's my guiding word again? Why can't I seem to feel that feeling?" "Amy explains it so clearly, I don't understand why it doesn't work for me. I know God tells me that I can do all things through Christ who strengthens me, but that must not apply to this because I'm confused and lost. Now I just want to eat. See, this is totally biological! My body is craving this. My body hates me! It's constantly working against me. *This* is why I can't lose weight!"

I promise you that you will most likely experience part, if not all, of these thoughts at some point in time. These thoughts are going to lead you to feel a certain way—frustrated, confused, angry, sad, and unmotivated. Guess what? You are normal, so take a long, deep breath. Make yourself a cup of tea and relax. You are just like the rest of us.

Your brain thinking these thoughts is totally normal. How do I know? My brain thinks them too. The reason it is normal for your brain to think this way is because it has been conditioned to. Now, before you get all confused and think, *How can I change, then, if my brain is just wired this way?*, read that sentence again. Your brain has been *conditioned* to think like this. You have practiced and practiced at thinking and responding in the way that you do. It is *easy*, and your brain *loves* easy.

Our brains are wired to be efficient. You have practiced beating yourself up, thinking in negative patterns, and believing that losing weight is hard, that food controls you, and that you are just meant to struggle with your weight. Because you have spent so much time practicing this pattern of thinking, your brain will go to these thoughts faster than I can inhale a cupcake sitting at a red light. The piece of the puzzle that might shock you is that your brain is causing you to feel frustrated, angry, sad, and hungry, even when you really are not. Now, before you get all ticked off at your brain, it is just doing what you have trained it to do; and to be fair, you probably were not intentionally training it to be so mean, but that is kind of what happened. At some point in your life, you began thinking in certain ways that caused you to feel certain feelings. The thing is, though, that you think the situation you are in is what is making you feel the way you feel, but it is not. The fact that you just started a new weight loss plan is not the reason you feel deprived. The fact that cookies are in the pantry is not actually what is causing your craving for them. The fact that your husband misunderstood your conversation about dinner is not the reason you are now wanting pizza. Your desire for food is caused by how you are choosing to think about the situation, not the situation itself.

Please, let this fact sink in. I know you may want to argue with me or give me all the reasons why your husband really *is* to blame for you eating pizza tonight, but he is not. I know that you fully believe that your body *has* to have cookies because they are within ten feet of you, but it does not. I know that you think your new eating plan *is* the sole cause of the fact that you feel like you have to white-knuckle it when the free donuts are calling your name at church, but it is not. The reason that you are eating pizza for dinner is because you are choosing to think about your husband not listening to you in a way that makes you want to eat pizza. The reason why you are craving the cookies is because you are thinking about them in a way that makes you desire to eat them. The reason why you want to shove those donuts in your mouth as fast (and discreetly) as possible is because you think *xyz*. Your thoughts about a certain fact are 100 percent responsible for how you feel about that fact, not the fact itself.

My client Debbie just celebrated her birthday. She struggled for two weeks leading up to that day because she knew her best friend was going to bake her a homemade Italian crème cake. The friend makes Debbie this cake every year, and it is her absolute favorite cake. Debbie had been working hard on her mind-set around food and had really started making the connection with the role she allowed food to play in her life. She had struggled in the past with overeating out of boredom, sadness, discomfort, joy, celebration, etc. You name the emotion, and Debbie would eat because of it. She had come quite a long way in making this connection with the action of overeating and was experiencing progress in stopping the use of food for emotions, but this birthday cake was really throwing her for a loop. She just could not imagine having the whole cake in her house. She just knew that she would eat it all. She considered asking her friend not to make her the cake. Then she thought about asking the friend to bring her only one slice or maybe bring the cake over only on the day of her birthday so she could share it with her family, as long as her friend would take the remainder of the cake when she left. Debbie just could not trust herself around the cake. Does this resonate with you? Do you struggle with having certain foods around you that feel like a trigger?

You may hate me for this, but the struggle is not about the food. The food has absolutely no control over you—you only think it does. The reason you cannot trust yourself around certain "trigger foods" is because you *think* that the food controls you. You keep telling yourself that food has control over you, that you love it so much, that it just tastes so good, etc. These thoughts are just that—thoughts. They are not facts, but you believe them. The result is that you eat the food, and you prove to yourself, then, that you were right.

When you can make the connection between your thoughts and your feelings and fully accept that your thoughts are a choice, you can break the cycle of emotional eating, deprivation, and lack of control. This connection was truly life-changing for me. I had to identify the story that I continued to tell myself about my struggle with food and how that played into the actions that I took. By identifying that story, I was finally able to understand why the cycle of emotional eating continued, because I believed that the struggle was a fact that could not be changed. Once I realized I could choose a new way to look at everything, then I could change the story. Then I could choose new thoughts.

Sometimes, though, your brain has a really hard time separating fact from fiction. A fact as defined by Merriam-Webster is "something that truly exists or happens, a situation or circumstance that is indisputable." I want to refer back to the childhood story I had created about my parents being divorced and being raised in the Catholic faith. The facts are my parents got divorced, and I went to a Catholic school and church. That is it. The story I created around these two facts are what led to my pain, confusion, and struggle. Now, I do not beat myself up for this story. I eventually realized that my thoughts had created this drama and that I had the ability to change my perspective and begin to heal from it. The facts are that lots of people's parents get divorced, and lots of kids are raised Catholic. I am sure many people have a similar story to mine, but just as many have a different one. The perspective (thoughts) that we bring to the facts is what creates the story, and our ability to not only recognize this but also choose how we want to reflect on a situation is essential for being intentional about our lives.

I could have continued to look at the facts of my life with disappointment, frustration, and despair; but to do that would have continued to leave me feeling the same way I was thinking. Then I would have acted out of those feelings. You and I have the choice to look at the facts of a situation and choose how we are going to interpret them. I now look at the fact that my parents divorced and understand that I did nothing wrong there. Everything happened exactly as it was supposed to for me. My Catholic faith was a solid foundation upon which to build my own personal relationship with God. It allowed me to learn, challenge my thoughts, and choose for myself what I wanted to believe. We all have this choice. The perspective or experience of a certain situation will be different for each person because every individual's thoughts are different. The facts of the situation may be the same, but the way we think about them will be different, and the thoughts will lead to how we feel about that experience.

Why is understanding this concept so important? It is not just so we can have a better understanding of how our brains work and how that directly affects our feelings, but it is so we can fully understand what typically happens from that place of feeling. Then, we will be able to identify the actions we take because of that feeling. For us emotional eaters, we tend to eat because of certain feelings (or all of the feelings). When we can make the connection between the thinking and feelings behind the action, we can finally have control over what we always thought was just a flaw. The fact that we lose and gain the same weight over and over again is not because we are just really bad at weight loss, it is because we are acting out in a way that we have thought, to this point, we did not have control over.

Let us go back to Debbie and the cake. The facts of the story are Debbie had a birthday, and her friend baked her a cake. Those are the facts, but Debbie created a whole story around what being in possession of the cake would mean, what might happen if she was left alone with the cake, and how she could not trust herself to not eat the whole cake. These were all just Debbie's thoughts, and her thoughts about the fact that her friend was bringing a cake led her to experience a ton of anxiety and worry. And guess what happened when Debbie felt anxious and worried? She ate. The fact is that Debbie was thinking about the cake in a way that led her to feel anxious and worried. The cake did not do that to her. In fact, the cake was not even in her possession when all of this worrying was happening. What Debbie was struggling with was seeing that the way she was choosing to think about the cake was causing all of her feelings.

Most of us have the same problem. We are not used to observing what our thoughts are and how they are controlling our feelings. We tend to look at a situation and think that *it* is what is driving our emotions. This makes us feel powerless because we cannot control all of our circumstances. You can control your thoughts, though, and your ability to choose your thoughts from a place of intention will directly impact the results you experience in your weight loss journey. This is where the application of your guiding word and Bible verse actually has impact. This is how Pam was able to make decisions from a place of peace to reach her healthy goals. She applied the knowledge and understanding of how her thoughts and feelings were connected to the decisions she makes.

This skill takes practice. If this is completely new knowledge to you, please, be patient with yourself and understand that success will come with practice and application. Look for some opportunities to start trying this out in small ways. Imagine that you are at the grocery store and that you are suddenly standing in front of a free sample of cookies. They are your favorite cookies. You used to eat them all of the time. You love how they taste, but you are not necessarily hungry. How could you look at this situation (your favorite cookie is in front of your face and *free*) in two different ways? I am going to assume an easy thought for you may be, *I love these cookies*, which leaves you wanting the cookie. Maybe, though, you do not want to desire the cookie. How could you think about the free cookie in such a way that you would have no desire for the cookie? This is when you have to try different thoughts out and see what works for you. Maybe by imagining that someone has sneezed on the cookie or by thinking that a bug has been on the cookie you can get rid of the desire. Maybe you can control the desire by just telling yourself you can have one later.

Going back to Debbie and the birthday cake one last time, I would have no issue if that cake sat in my house all weekend long, and that is not because I have some amazing superpower now that protects me from the desire of sweet, yummy goodness. I have an allergy to dairy; therefore, I would never knowingly eat that cake because I have thoughts that dairy will make me feel horrible for four days, so I do not eat it.

The only difference between Debbie and me with regards to the cake is our thoughts about the cake.

You can have that kind of victory, too. You can choose to look at food, weight loss, and your healthy goals in a way that leaves you feeling empowered, not deprived; capable, not lacking; and motivated, not a failure. I love that not only does science back all of this up, but God speaks on it too. In Romans 12:2, He calls us to be transformed by the renewing of our minds. Understanding this truth and aligning your thoughts with God, my friends, is how you can actually have victory.

The next time you find yourself overwhelmed with unwanted emotions, stop and ask yourself these questions:

- What are the facts of the situation? (Remember, facts are indisputable.)
- What are my thoughts about the situation? (Pretty much everything else going on in your mind.)
- How do these thoughts make me feel? (Use one-word answers: angry, sad, happy, afraid, joyful.)
- When I feel this way, what do I usually do? What actions do I take?
- What are the results of these actions?

When you start to connect the dots of how your thoughts drive your feelings, and your feelings drive your actions, and your actions dictate the results, you will see not only why you have the results that you do in your life but also how to intentionally make different choices to achieve your most desired goals.

~Change your thoughts,
change your life.

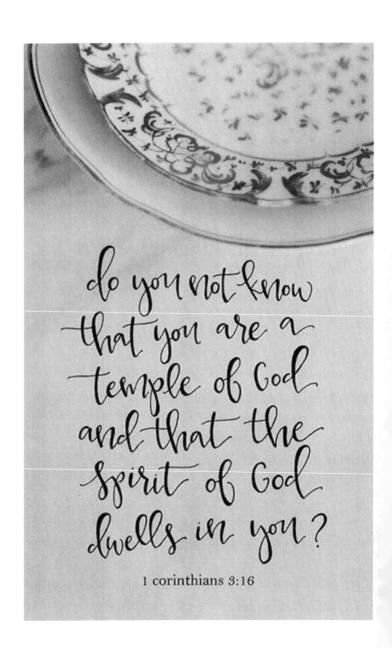

do you not know that you are a temple of God and that the spirit of God dwells in you?

1 corinthians 3:16

Chapter 4: Learning to Listen to Your Body

You are conditioned to wanting a meal plan to start a new diet; to counting calories to lose weight; and to eating breakfast, lunch, and dinner at certain times of the day regardless of whether you are hungry. You think and are told that this is the way to eat healthy, lose weight, and stop overeating. You try to follow the instructions, but you eventually get tired of it all. None of it really addresses who you are as an individual, what you are experiencing, and what you go through with food. The diets and plans do not consider how you feel when you are hungry or what your body's reactions are to certain foods. The diet industry perpetuates the thought that you cannot listen to your body, that you are not smart enough to make decisions on your own, and that you cannot trust yourself.

All of this is pretty easy for you to buy into because you have thought the same thing your whole life, right? You can replay all the times you have tried your hardest to diet and failed. Every single pound you have lost and gained back is clear in your mind and only proves to you that you are a failure and cannot trust yourself. You can easily believe that you need to override your body's cues because it does not know what it is talking about anyway, right?

Well, my friend, I am offering you a chance at freedom from this struggle. You no longer have to believe that you are incapable of figuring out and deciding what works best for your body. You get to take back control over something you may have thought you never had control over to begin with. Now is the time to rebuild this relationship with your body, to reconnect, and to become friends.

Friendship seems really hard to have with something that you feel never worked right for you from the beginning, something that could not be trusted, and something that was just waiting to prove you wrong. These reasons are why your current relationship with your body borders more on forced tolerance than love and why you cringe when you read or hear Bible verses that remind you that your body is the temple of the Holy Spirit, that you are not your own, that your body was bought and paid for with the blood of Christ (I Cor. 6:19-20). These verses only makes you feel *worse* about yourself, not better or in the least bit motivated.

The disconnect with your body continues. You continue to buy into the notion that a better diet is out there waiting for you. If you just count so many calories, fat grams, carbs, and macros a day, you will lose all the weight you want. You know from experience that these diets do work for a short time. You can, and have, lost weight following them all. Only, you end up gaining it back when that "plan" does not work for you anymore.

Have a moment of true honesty here, my friend. The diets *do* work. You will lose weight doing them as long as you keep doing them, right? Where the diet "fails" is when you no longer want to follow the plan. You no longer want to log every point that goes into your mouth. Diets cease to "work" because we choose not to live the rest of our lives according to a diet (which is what is required to keep the weight off).

Listen, I am all for losing unwanted weight, and I am all for filling our bodies with tasty and nutritious food, but another way to do this exists. It requires something that you may have never tried before in your weight loss journey. It requires patience, love, and commitment to listening to what your body's hunger needs are and then fulfilling that need. Please, read that again.

Your body has hunger needs, and food was designed to fulfill those needs—nothing more. Food was never meant to help you feel better emotionally. Food can only solve one problem: physical hunger. The process of learning to connect to and make decisions from a place of your body's true signals and needs is a different level of losing weight. It is a natural way—intuitive even.

I help my clients identify their body's fuel needs by using a tool called the hunger scale. This tool was taught to me by my life coach and weight loss instructor, Brooke Castillo. Imagine a scale starting at a negative ten and going to a positive ten with zero in the middle. A negative ten would be absolutely starving, past the point of hanger (you know, hunger + anger), and a positive ten is stuffed, almost physically sick. The zero in the middle represents a neutral state. Food is not even on your radar screen. I guide my clients to learn to eat when they are around a negative two of hunger and to stop when they hit a positive two on the scale. Figuring out what your body's signals are for these levels takes a little practice. Each person has individual cues that his or her body gives him or her to determine what his or her true hunger level is.

Here is an example. Lilly spent her life going through different phases of dieting, from starting a new diet to no dieting to another new diet. She lost and gained the same sixty pounds more times than she could count. Several times in her life she ate so sparingly that her body's natural responses shut down, she experienced hair loss, and her periods stopped. Even when she was at her lowest weight, she was obsessed with keeping it all off. She completely lost touch with her body and only used it as an instrument that she could control when everything else was out of control. When she came to me, she was at one of her highest weights again in her life and feeling defeated. She was close to giving up on ever being able to really lose the weight. We started working together and making progress on the mind-set connection with her weight struggles. I introduced to her the hunger scale, and she began learning what her body's responses were to true hunger as well as satisfaction. These were really new ideas to her because she was so used to diets that went from periods of white-knuckle hunger to binging on forbidden foods until she was so full her stomach hurt.

She started to recognize her cue of a negative two hunger as rumbling in her stomach, a desire to eat, but not to a level of hangry. At this level, she knew that if she ate now and stopped at a positive two she would be sustained for at least another four hours or so, when her body would start to signal hunger again. She was finding comfort in acknowledging the negative two as a sign to eat and no longer depended on the clock or time of day to decide her eating plan for her. She was still working on finding the comfort at stopping at a positive two, where her body was nutritionally satisfied. She would tell me that at the positive two level, she was satisfied, her stomach was not too full, and she could fairly easily go out for a walk without feeling physically uncomfortable from the food in her stomach. Her struggle was with the mental desire to keep eating. This was a new way of life for her, and it required her attention each time she ate.

She found in the beginning that not having distractions around her (no phone or TV) when she ate was best and that stopping at certain times to check in with her body was a good way for her to know at what level she was. She also found that her body would naturally sigh when she was right about at that positive two level. That sigh was a good indicator that one or two more bites was all her body really needed to have the fuel it required for the next few hours. The *desire* to eat more was still there at times, though. Sometimes she could easily stop at the positive two and be done—no stress, no drama. At other times, her mind wanted more. She would tell herself that she should not waste the food that was left. Sometimes, the food was just so good that she did not want to stop.

This mental chatter that happens when your body is nutritionally satisfied, but your mind is not, is quite common for emotional eaters who are learning to eat intuitively. Up until this point, you have probably been completely disconnected from what your body's true physiological needs are and what your mind is telling you it wants. This is not a bad thing or indicative of your ability to eat from a place of honoring your body. This is actually a good sign of what to address from the standpoint of *why* you emotionally eat. As I explained in the "intentional thoughts" chapter, your thoughts are directly connected to your feelings of desire to continue eating past the level of your body's needs. When your mind is saying, "This food is so good. I don't want to stop eating it," your mind is being efficient at thinking what you have practiced telling yourself for years. It is using the well-paved road of thought around what role food is playing in your life.

I hope we can agree on this point. If you are eating *more* than what your body is telling you it needs, you are then using food for something more than fuel. You are at this point using food for some emotional reason. The key to being able to stop emotional eating is to recognize when you are doing it and why. Being able to connect to your body's hunger needs is essential to beginning the recognition process. Once you are able to identify where your hunger is on a scale, you will be able to begin addressing your reasons for overeating.

Another client, Tammie, struggled over the years with emotional eating. She had tried controlling her overeating by cutting out certain food groups, limiting the types of foods that she ate, and only eating what she had deemed "healthy." Still, she overate. Her desire to eat healthy foods was met, she was at a manageable weight, but she still struggled with overeating, which kept her from reaching her body's natural weight. Even though Tammie had addressed the types of foods that worked well for her body, she was still using food for emotional reasons. I had her start journaling her food—no calorie counting. The journal's purpose was to help her identify *why* she was overeating. Each time she ate past a positive two, she described what was going on for her at that moment, what thoughts were coming up for her, and what was driving her desire to continue eating.

This is where being open to the learning process of listening to your body is essential. You are rebuilding a relationship with yourself. Remember, up to this point your source of connection with your body has been distrust, frustration, sadness, and anger. Now, you are building a relationship that allows you to not only listen to your body's feedback but to also make decisions from a place of honor from that feedback. Your body has been talking to you for years, asking you to listen, and actually gaining weight while trying to get your attention. Maybe instead of weight gain, it has been acting out in the form of constipation, bloating, indigestion heartburn, headaches, or sickness. It wants you to connect with it and respect what it needs and deserves. I love the quote by Nayyirah Waheed that says, "And I said to my body. Softly. I want to be your friend. It took a long breath. And replied, 'I have been waiting my whole life for this.'"

I'm not going to tell you that this journey will be easy, but you are worth figuring it out. You are worth learning to listen to and honoring your body. You are worth identifying why you want to overeat. You are worth the commitment to understanding how your mind is connected to your desire to overeat. You are worth the reminder that you are in control of your thoughts and that you have the power and ability to stop yourself in the action of overeating. You are capable of ending this cycle my friend, and ending it starts with listening to and connecting with your body.

Commit to rebuilding a relationship with your body from a judgement-free zone. Recognize the story you tell yourself about why you are overweight, why diets do not work for you, and why you emotionally eat. Recognize how this story makes you feel. Are you ready to feel differently? Are you willing to challenge your past thinking and rewrite your story? What do you need to tell yourself to give yourself permission to make this change and connection?

Download free worksheet to help you start eating based on your body's hunger needs and asking your body the best questions for feedback.

www.losethementalweight.com/listentoyourbody

~Listen to your body. It is always communicating with you.

Chapter 5: How to Feel Your Feelings and Stop Eating Them

Do you remember a time you were standing in the kitchen, emotions surging, and feeling frantic? All you could think about was food. You did not even know if you were hungry or not. The desire to eat just felt so strong. You headed to the refrigerator to scan the contents. *What's in here that sounds good? Anything in the freezer?* You walked over to the pantry and took inventory. *There are some chips, a few cookies, some healthier snacks.* You had purposefully not bought a lot of your yummy treats because you were trying so hard not to overeat. You thought that not having your trigger foods in the house would work. You grabbed the bag of healthy granola. *This isn't bad. I'll just have a little of this*. You ate some and put it back. Then you stood there looking, searching for something else. You did not feel satisfied. *What else sounds good?* You grabbed the sunflower seeds. *These are good for me. They won't hurt*. You poured out some into a bowl thinking to yourself, *at least I'm not just sitting here zoned out and eating them by the handful*. You sat down and slowly ate through the sunflower seeds, but then they were gone.

Now what? you thought to yourself. *I'm still "hungry." I'm still not satisfied.* So you headed back to the kitchen and looked for the next snack item. Before you knew it, you had snacked on several different items, maybe to the point of discomfort, and then you were beating yourself up. Once again, the idea of being healthy took a total backseat to the little gremlin inside you that just wanted food. The feelings just feel so overwhelming at times. They seem to just come out of nowhere. You did *so* well all week, but now you feel like a complete failure. Food won again. *Why do I keep doing this?* you ask.

We have all been there. As an emotional eater, the desire for food has won over the desire we have to lose weight many times. Sometimes we can string together a few weeks of honoring whatever diet we have put ourselves on, but the urge to eat continues, and sometimes we just give in. Understanding where this desire comes from is key in unlocking how to stop this cycle. Looking back on the scenario I just laid out, can you see that the hunger for more food was not a true physical hunger? It did not originate from your body telling you that it needed fuel. It was your mind. Your mind was hungry.

A good indicator of whether what you are experiencing is mental hunger or physical hunger is if you would be "satisfied" by sitting down and having a "normal" snack or meal. When the urge to eat is so strong, would an apple and peanut butter be enough, or would you find yourself back in the kitchen searching for more? This is when listening to your body's true physiological feedback is going to help you identify true hunger, and what you have been practicing throughout the week of dialing into that hunger will help you to be able to identify this specific hunger when your mind wants more.

The intense cravings you experience that cannot be satisfied by a normal snack are just emotional responses to whatever you are thinking at that moment. If your body has what it needs to function, your desire to eat is coming solely from your mind. The feelings that you might not even be able to name in the moment (the ones surging through your body that feel so uncomfortable you just want to distract yourself from them) are just your reaction to a thought. They feel like so much more than that, but that is typically because we have never taken the time to truly acknowledge them or honor them.

Have you ever just allowed yourself to feel angry, sad, anxious, or worried without acting on the emotion? Have you ever processed how these emotions feel and named them? Most of the time we are pretty quick to say when we are mad, but do you sit with it, feel it, and become aware of what you are thinking that is causing the anger? Or do you go off about it, yell as a result of it, or call your mom or best friend and tell them all the details of why you are so angry? Because whether you are yelling, venting, or stuffing food into your mouth, you are taking actions from this place of emotion, and you do not have to.

Emotions and feelings are really not the big, scary, overwhelming, nonnegotiable things that we think they are. They are just a product of our thinking. Whatever emotion you are feeling at a certain time is directly connected to what you are thinking in the moment. Let us use an easy emotion to start with as an example. When I graduated from high school and walked across the stage, my mom was proud, happy, and excited for me. Most parents would be, right? Well, that is not necessarily true. The act of graduating and walking across a stage does not automatically result in parents feeling proud, happy, or excited. The reason my mom felt this way was because she was thinking about things that made her feel this way. Maybe she was thinking about how far I had come since becoming a teenager or how hard she had worked to help raise me or what my future might look like as I headed off to college. Her thinking on these things (or whatever she was actually thinking) is what led to the happy emotions.

I am pretty sure that not all parents were feeling that way that day. I know some who were disappointed because their child was choosing to do things with his or her life with which the parents did not agree. I know some parents were sad to see their children grow up and leave. Some parents were angry because they were currently fighting with the rest of the family that had come to graduation that day. I chose this example because it is probably so far removed from what you are experiencing when you are sitting at home trying not to eat. Hopefully, you can see that the emotion is caused by a person's perception (which, according to Merriam Webster's dictionary, is "the way an individual thinks about or understands something") of a situation.

Many times, seeing how someone else's thoughts about a particular situation are his or her choice is easier than seeing the same thing about our own. When we are looking at our own reactions in a particular moment, remembering that they are our choice is not so simple because our emotions feel so real and so intense. Wrapping our brains around the fact that those deep, dark feelings that seem to be so overwhelming in the moment are actually within our control is hard. They are not the abyss that we fear so much. They are not the dangerous landmine that we are trying so hard to avoid. Feelings, on their own, are not dangerous. The danger comes when we act from those feelings. Feelings, as my teacher likes to describe them, are just sensations in our bodies that result from a thought in our head—period.

What makes the feelings seem so intense is the perpetual cycle of the thoughts causing them. When the feelings are too intense, we want to run away from them. The last thing we want to do in the moment is embrace them, si* with them, and feel them; but that is where your freedom lies. Your ability to overcome emotional eating resides solely in your willingness to actually process your feelings and stop running from them, stop eating them, stop denying them, stop acting them out, stop yelling at your spouse, and stop venting about them to whoever will listen. Just feel them, process them, and acknowledge them. From this place, you will be able to take back from them the ability to be responsible and to make decisions that honor yourself and your goals. You will be able to show up in the world exactly how you most desire too, without regret.

I am working with Terry on her ability to process her emotions of anger at her husband without numbing them with food. Terry struggles with the fact that her husband thinks so differently from her on how they should react to their family. He has a very detached relationship when it comes to responding to things going on with his parents and siblings, and it drives Terry crazy. She thinks he needs to be more involved. She thinks he needs to speak his mind more and not let them run all over him and call the shots with everything. She has tried making suggestions to her husband on how to handle these situations, but he has not done anything to change it. Terry gets very frustrated; and when something specific happens, she feels put out by it all. She just wants a distraction. She decides to treat herself to chocolate and wine. She laughs and tells me, "What's life without chocolate and wine? I don't care if I'm thinner or not. These are my friends! They save my sanity! These keep me from just losing it on my husband and telling him exactly how I feel." I know that Terry really does not want to numb out, but she is also fearful of feeling her anger and having to own the fact that she is creating it. Struggling with the food and weight feel so much more desirable to her.

Until she is willing to feel a new kind of uncomfortable by processing these emotions and owning her thoughts about her husband, that struggle will continue.

You see, we really do not need anyone or anything else to change in order for us to change. We think we need our husbands, our kids, our parents, or our siblings to get their act together and work on improving themselves before we can feel better. We believe that our feelings are tied to their actions, but they do not have to be. Believe it or not, our ability to process and work through emotions is only directly connected to someone, or something, else if we make it. If you choose to go that route, then own the fact that you have handed over your feelings to someone else. You have given up responsibility for yourself to someone else. You have chosen the role of victim, and, sadly, making the changes that you want to in life from this place is going to be really hard.

True change requires you to own who you are and the role you play in your life and to take responsibility for how you think, feel, and react. Think about this truth for a second. Do you not want for your husband, kids, parents, etc., to take responsibility for how they think, feel, and react? Is that not what you *really* want them to do, but you are not willing to do so yourself?

Terry wants so badly for her husband to act differently with his family, but she is not willing to act differently in response to her own emotions. She is struggling with feeling her own discomfort with her emotions so much that she eats chocolate and drinks wine and then blames her husband for not doing things differently. She is stuck thinking that he has to do something different for her to be able to. The point she is missing in this struggle is that if she allows herself to process the feelings of anger and frustration and connects them to what she *thinks* her husband needs to do, she can actually take authority over the emotions. This position requires her to quit looking outside of herself for better feelings, though, and to quit abdicating control over her emotions and actions to someone else. When she is willing to acknowledge her thoughts about her husband and process the emotions that come up for her, she will be able to stop turning to food and alcohol to make her feel differently.

You are doing the same thing when you turn to food (or other distractions) impulsively in the moment you want to feel differently. You may not even be able to identify what emotion you are experiencing—you just want it to stop. You want the feeling to go away. Feelings do not just go away on their own, though. Even in the act of eating, you are just replacing one feeling with another. You are simply acting in a way that will lead you to feel different emotions.

Typically, the numbing feeling is only temporary. Eventually, you then feel a different emotion based on what you are thinking when you are in that moment of distraction or shortly thereafter. When you are done distracting yourself with food, feelings of disgust, disappointment, and shame come to light. Those feelings are directly connected to what you are saying to yourself when you are present and aware again. When you put the food down and are physically stuffed, the thoughts turn to, *Why did I do that? That didn't help, anyway. I'm just a mess*. Eating for a feeling is just a vicious cycle, my friends, and the only way to stop it is to own it.

One of the exercises I walk my clients through is being able to identify their emotions: name them, feel them, describe them, and then journal about what they are telling themselves about this certain situation. What story have they created? After they have separated the facts from the story, I encourage them to sit down in a quiet space and process everything. This is uncomfortable at times, but you can do uncomfortable. When you are willing to sit with yourself with this level of awareness, honesty, and maturity, you will be able to make the connection and stop emotionally eating. You will be able to better identify each impulse as it happens. You will be able to stop yourself in that moment, to choose differently, and to let go of the weight you no longer want to carry, not only the physical weight but also the mental weight that shows up in your food struggles.

Download free worksheets to begin learning how to identify and process your feelings.

www.losethementalweight.com/feelyourfeelings

~Feelings are just visitors, let them come and go.

Chapter 6: Movement as Praise

Do you have a love/hate relationship with exercise? Do you find yourself enjoying it sometimes and feeling like it is a burden at others? What role does exercise play in your life? Do you still see it as a way to burn a ton of calories, to punish yourself for eating poorly, or to beat your body into submission?

If you are currently viewing exercise as anything other than a way to cherish and care for the body you currently have, the fact that you hate exercising is no small wonder. I know the world tells us all the newest ways to burn calories, to get the best-looking legs, and to lose weight fast with new types of workouts and exercise plans. Granted, exercise can do some of these things, but it is just a small piece of the puzzle, and keeping it in the current role of bully/torture/punishment typically will not help you to make exercise your new BFF.

Consequently, I often hear from clients, "I know I need to work out, but (1) I just don't have the time, (2) I just don't feel like it, or (3) I just don't like it." If you struggle consistently with making exercise a part of your life because of these three reasons, I can help you.

The first reason I hear for not exercising is the time factor, and it is always a big reason. Generally, those who use it have tons of evidence to back up the reason, too. They work fifty-plus hours a week; their kids are busy with other activities; the where/when of how they want to work out just does not fit into their schedule. I know these reasons may feel like truth to you, but they are just your thoughts and the way you are choosing to look at the situation. If exercise (movement) is important to you, you will carve out time for it in your schedule. It will become a priority to you just like brushing your teeth, keeping an appointment, or paying your taxes. It will become a nonnegotiable.

A lot of times, though, exercise fails to be a priority because of the role you give it in your life. If you truly see it as something like punishment, of course you will put it on the backburner and not make it something you pencil into your calendar just like every other appointment. In fact, it will actually become something you try to avoid. This may be the first time you have ever considered that exercise could play a different role in your life. You may have never before considered that exercise can actually be something you give to yourself or do from a place of gratitude, or even praise, for this life and the body with which you have been blessed.

The ideas that exercise can be an expression of gratitude and praise and that it can be something other than a means through which you burn calories can be difficult for some people to wrap their minds around at first, especially if you are still struggling with loving yourself as you are today. The ability to honor your body and care for it even when you still want to lose weight, though, is what is going to allow you to listen to your body's cues, to feel your feelings, and to move in a way that feels good to you. Beating your body into submission has not worked up until now (I know you have tried), so now is the perfect time for a different approach. Let us vow, from this moment forward, to see the gift of life we have been given in this body; the blessing of being able to move, breathe, and sweat; and the joy we can find in honoring ourselves each and every day. From this place of honor, you will see that exercise is something you do *for* your body, not *to* your body; and just as you decided at some point that brushing your teeth was important to your health, you can make that same decision about exercise. It can become a nonnegotiable in your schedule as well.

My client Susy had a full-time job as a manager over her entire department. She was divorced with two kids, and her schedule was full, to say the least. She knew that exercise was important to her overall health but just could not see how she was supposed to fit one more activity into her life. She beat herself up and felt guilty for the fact that she did not do it, but also held tightly to her beliefs that she just did not have time for it. She used to exercise; she would go to classes after work. She had even found that she enjoyed the kickboxing and spinning classes. When life changed, however, and she got divorced, stopping on her way home from work for those classes just did not fit her new life; so she quit exercising all together. Now she wanted to lose some of the weight she had put on since her divorce and could not figure out how to get back into exercise.

We talked a lot about what role she saw exercise playing in her weight loss journey. She felt like she could not lose weight unless she was burning as many calories as possible, four nights a week. She was also new to my approach of eating based off of her hunger scale and was skeptical of how all of this was going to work, so we talked about looking at exercise a little differently in her plan. We discussed how she could view exercise in a way that freed her to find movement that not only fit into her schedule but also allowed her to make it a priority in her overall health, not just a method of burning calories. She was open to trying out some different approaches and thought it would be helpful if she found some ways to move that actually helped reduce her stress and allowed her the ability to reconnect with her mind and body. She knew part of the reason she had gained weight since her divorce was because she had gone into survival mode and put herself on the back burner. She began by deciding how many times a week (and for how long) she would commit to movement, whether it was a walk at lunch, yoga in the morning, or a workout class on the weekend, no matter what was going on in her schedule. She decided that exercise needed to be a part of her life, and she realized that the only way to accomplish this goal was to make it nonnegotiable by making it a priority for both her physical health and mental health.

If you want exercise to play this type of role in your life, you will need to do the same. Decide that no matter what, movement is important enough to your mental, physical, and spiritual health that it will be a priority on your schedule. Decide what your minimum commitment is to exercise. It can be for however many days and however much time to which you will commit; but once you decide what works best for you, it goes on to your schedule just like any other appointment. You place it there not because you cannot trust yourself to exercise but because you have decided that movement is important enough to you to make it a priority in your life.

The second stumbling block I see with my clients and exercise is lack of motivation. I hear many of them say, "I just don't feel like exercising." Many times, lack of motivation happens when you are stuck in the viewpoint of exercise being something that you *have* to do and not something that you *choose* to do. You will have days when your energy is low, and you may need to take a rest day or do something that requires less energy. Listening to and honoring your body's feedback and actually taking those days of rest when your body is telling you it needs one is important, but be willing to dig a little deeper into that, "I don't wanna," and understanding fully from where this thought is originating is equally important. Is it coming from a place of true physical exhaustion or illness, or is it coming from a lack of desire?

Understanding that your mind can dictate your feelings is huge in addressing not only your desires to emotionally eat but also understanding when you do not desire to care for yourself. That sounds harsh, I know, but on some level you have to recognize the relationship between the struggle of not fully "wanting" to take care of yourself and love yourself and the struggle that goes directly to whatever story you are telling yourself in that moment. When you do, you can get clear on what the facts of the situation are and what story you may be creating around the struggle.

Susy is a great example of this. She struggled with the desire to make herself a priority again after her divorce. She slowly started to uncover the story she had created around her worthiness and the hurt, sadness, and pain that she had not fully processed from the end of her marriage. Because of those feelings, putting herself at the bottom of the priority list because of the kids and her schedule was easy. This really happened, though, because she no longer saw herself as important. She had a lot of unrecognized thoughts and feelings about what her divorce meant to her, and without even being aware of it, she was placing the blame on herself, believing that she was not good enough, worthy enough, or deserving enough of love. Because she thought all of these things were true as a result of her husband leaving her, she no longer felt like she was worthy enough of her own love and attention. These were not decisions of which she was fully aware; but because she was subconsciously thinking and feeling this way, her physical, mental, and spiritual health were suffering. Feeding and moving her body in a way that was nourishing no longer felt like something that really mattered because deep down she did not feel like she mattered anymore. Understanding what was driving Susy's lack of desire was tied to her understanding those lingering thoughts and feelings about what had happened in her life.

A lack of desire to care for and honor yourself with your food and movement choices is typically grounded in thoughts you have around whether caring for yourself matters anyways, whether you are worthy of your own attention and love, and what the purpose of everything is. This is where reevaluating your *why* will be important along your journey. Getting clear on why you choose to love and honor yourself with your choices will help clear the path when things get foggy. Remember your value and your worth as defined by God. He chose you, He formed your perfectly in your mother's womb (Ps. 139:13–16). He delights in you (Ps. 139:17–18). He sent His Son for you (Rom. 5:8). Many of our past thoughts and beliefs will still come up from time to time; but as you continue to make the connection between God's love for you and how you should value yourself, you will take back control over what is important to you and will not allow fleeting moments of distraction take you off course.

The third reason I often hear is, "I just don't like to exercise." A part of making exercise a priority in your life is finding ways to move that you actually enjoy. I know "exercise" and "enjoy" do not always go together in your brain

They did not in mine either, but as you now know, thoughts can change! Again, I think the old thoughts of exercise being something that we do *to* our bodies instead of *for* our bodies tend to trip us up with being okay with choosing to workout in ways that we actually like.

The habit of thinking of exercise as a weight loss tool leads us to look at what workouts will whip us into shape instead of workouts that we actually enjoy and feel good doing. Now, "enjoying" and "feel good doing" do not always mean "not challenging" or "easy." Choosing things that feel easier to you is definitely okay. In the beginning, staying open to feelings of discomfort when you are figuring out what you like is a good idea. Stepping out of your comfort zone will be required to try new things, but eventually, you may find that your favorite way to exercise is a class that is actually hard and challenges you. You may find that you enjoy the feeling, or you may find that you feel your best when you are moving in a way that feels comforting to you and sacred. There is no wrong way to move. Only you will be able to fully know what works best for you. Understand that what works best may change as you change; you may go through seasons where you actually enjoy harder, more strenuous exercise and other times walking and gentle yoga will fill you up fully! This is the joy of deciding what works best for you and of being open to that changing, which can feel scary and uncertain at times if you are thinking your exercise choices should be made by you comparing your healthy definition to someone else's. Understand that what works for you may not work for the next person and vice versa.

God did not create all of us exactly the same. He created us each unique and different because we all have a specific purpose and path. Ultimately, He wants us to lean on

Him in each moment for support, strength, and guidance and then reflect the source of your light out to others. Keep these truths in mind if you find yourself questioning your current exercise plan. Make sure you are choosing workouts that work well for you in the current season of your life. Allow yourself the freedom to explore and change your ideas about exercise in a way that feels loving, nourishing, and healthy to you.

- Make exercise a priority, a nonnegotiable, for you. Determine the minimum days per week and time per day of movement that will be on your schedule, no matter what.
- Be aware of the story you are creating around why you do not "feel" like exercising. Honor your body's true feedback and challenge your thoughts around why exercise is important to you.
- Find movement that you enjoy, with which you can connect, and that fills you up.

~Exercise to honor your body, not to punish it.

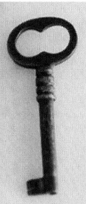

but the fruit of the spirit is love, joy, peace, patience, kindness, goodness, faithfulness, gentleness, self-control; against such things there is no law.

galatians 5: 22-23

Chapter 7: Applying God's Word

When you are searching for a quick start to weight loss or to cleanse your body of toxins or to stop overeating, can you identify what feeling is driving the search? Is it fear, frustration, sadness, disappointment, or anger? Usually, when we feel like we are struggling with emotional eating again and the weight has crept back on, we are not feeling our best, and we get stuck thinking, *If I can just jumpstart my weight loss, then I'll feel better.* Maybe you think, *If I can just find the RIGHT diet plan—this will finally work*, or you ask yourself, *Is something medically wrong with me that causes me to overeat and gain weight so easily?* These thoughts typically lead to feelings of desperation, and sometimes, that desperation leads to a new diet/exercise plan for us to try. Unfortunately, though, we still have not dealt with the mental junk we keep carrying around, so the new diet plan or cleanse only works for a short period of time. We are still left with the thoughts that led us to feeling frustrated, sad, desperate, and downtrodden in the first place.

At this point, I hope you have made the connection with how your thoughts often drive your feelings, and your feelings often drive your actions. For us emotional eaters, action usually involves food. Most of the time, eating is our way of numbing out or distracting ourselves from whatever emotion we are experiencing at that time. What that emotion is does not really matter, but if it feels intense or we feel thrown off by it, we eat.

Now that you know how to feel your feelings and how to stop being so afraid of them, the next step is to not only better understand where those feeling are coming from (your thoughts) but to also take ownership of them and recognize that *you* are in control of your thoughts. You have to recognize that the feelings that you want to feel so badly from that new diet or cleanse (peace, control, joy, comfort) are available to you right now, in this moment. You do not have to change anything about the specific circumstance or situation you are in. You just have to change your thoughts regarding it. This is how you attain the feeling you so desperately want. Your freedom from struggle comes from right thinking, so does control of your emotions.

For us Jesus Girls, we have the best source for those feelings of peace, love, acceptance, worthiness, and joy that we want so badly. We have God's truth written out for us in the Bible. Growing up Catholic, I did not spend a lot of time studying or memorizing Bible verses. Growing up in the South, I quickly figured out that I was "missing" something when my Southern Baptist friends could recite Bible verses like song lyrics. I was always caught a little off guard as to where they had learned them and why I was never taught how to "study" the Bible.

I did not let go of the judgement I felt toward myself and the embarrassment that I felt over not knowing how to "dig into" God's Word until my late thirties. I personally carried about the criticism regarding my worthiness to even speak about what the Bible said, so this Jesus Girl went and bought a study Bible and just started reading. Before that, my only personal relationship with the Bible was limited to randomly opening it for some hopes of an, "Aha!" moment when things were *really* bad. When whatever was going on at that moment (financial stress, an argument with my husband, family disagreements) felt *so* overwhelming it would literally drive me to my knees (and food), then I would grab my Bible and desperately search for some answer to what I was experiencing.

That study Bible was a new experience for this girl. I was so grateful for the notes section at the bottom of the verses that helped shine some light on the meaning behind language that I had a hard time understanding, much less applying to my current predicament. Slowly, but surely, I began to read God's Word with a curiosity that I had once only had for fiction. The more I began to "dig in," the more He revealed Himself to me as He promises in Jeremiah 29:13, "You will seek me and find me when you seek me with all of your heart." The more I began to speak to Him, the more He began to speak back; and no, not in an audible way; but in subtle signs that were enough for me to know that they were not some kind of coincidence. As I began acknowledging these signs as messages from Him, the more I was able to lean into His word, His truth, His love, and His promises for me (Proverbs 2:1–6).

As I continued practicing the understanding of my own feelings in relation to my thoughts, I began to recognize that the feelings I had been searching for were already available to me through His promises as a follower of Christ. I became aware of where my thinking was not in alignment with His Word, and then I could start to replace my thoughts with His truths. This is where His Word came to life for me. This is how I learned to actually apply the Bible to my everyday mess. Instead of frantically searching for a hidden message, I started using the Bible verses that spoke to me to replace my own thoughts and challenge the story I was creating about a situation.

Often, I think we struggle with how to apply a message

that is thousands of years old to what we are currently experiencing. By understanding the feeling that you want to have regarding whatever is happening, you can find the promises that He has already made to you; and then by choosing to believe Him in that moment, the feeling you truly want is there. When the struggle is real to actually *feel* the feeling God has promised, you know you have an opportunity to dig a little deeper and determine what lies you are believing at that time. As Jesus Girls, we have the choice to believe what God has promised us, or we can choose to let the world's views take over and leave us feeling lost, sad, and defeated. These are not feelings from God.

At this point our feelings are not only a good opportunity to stop and become aware of what we are telling ourselves but also a chance to examine those thoughts with God's Word. From this place of truth, when we choose to believe Him for His promises, we will finally experience the feelings we hope and pray will come from our next diet, exercise plan, or magical weight. Unfortunately, we get stuck thinking that all of these factors are what will finally bring us peace, joy, and happiness; but they will not by themselves. The good news is that you can start to feel these feelings now before anything else has to change by just changing your thoughts to reflect His truth.

Jeremiah 29:11 is one of my favorite Bible verses and was the first verse that I clung to when I was experiencing a long season of personal difficulties. "'For I know the plans I have for you,' says the Lord, 'plans to prosper you and not to harm you, plans to give you hope and a future.'" When this verse appeared in my life several years ago, I was going through some very tough times. I had lost both of my grandmother within a year of each other and then, very suddenly, lost my dad. To say these events rocked my world is an understatement. I truly felt like the things that had anchored me to the world had gone away. I felt off-balance, shaken, and unsure of what was coming next. At the same time, my husband was dealing with health issues, I had left my "secure" job to follow my passion, our economy was still a mess from the events of 2008, our income was slashed in half, and the market that drove my husband's industry was at a standstill. I honestly did not know what was going to happen from moment to moment. I felt like I was walking a tightrope that was about to snap in half.

I am not going to lie to you and tell you that I remember the exact day that God revealed Jeremiah 29:11 to me because I do not recall. He did, though, and He made sure to put the message in my heart. In those desperate times when my mind would start to run away from me, when I would feel the anxiety and worry taking over, I would repeat that Bible verse to myself over and over again. I clung to His promise of a plan for me and to this truth that His plans were to "prosper me and not to harm me, to give me a hope and a future." This was the first time that thirtysomething Jesus Girl had memorized a Bible verse in her life, and I had a choice in those moments. I could choose to believe Him for His promises, or not. The choice was mine.

The choice is yours, too. If you believe His Word as truth, then applying this truth to your life is the way to find the feelings you crave and to feel in control, joyful, and loved. He has bought and paid the price for you, and part of His amazing gift of salvation is the joy and peace you desire. As if eternal heaven with Him is not enough, He has given you the ability to experience some Heaven on Earth as well.

How does this apply to your weight loss journey? Well, it starts with a Bible verse, one that speaks to you and that God has put on your heart. What does this verse promise? Love? Worthiness? Peace? Joy? Provision? Strength? Do you believe this verse? When you believe this verse, do you feel that feeling, the one you described? Understand that this feeling may not come to you immediately, but this is how you start to apply His word to your thinking. When you are in a moment of unwanted emotion (anger, frustration, etc.), you can replace your thoughts with this verse. You meditate on it. You journal it. You connect with it and choose to believe it. Your feelings will change as you continue to meditate on the Word of God.

Next, I want you to clarify what actions you take when you are feeling unwanted emotions. What do you do when you feel that way? For most of us emotional eaters, eating is one of the actions which then leads to you "proving" your original negative thought. If at this point you can learn to lean into His Word instead of food, your relationship with food, yourself, and God will change. You will begin to store up His promises in your heart; and instead of heading to the pantry or refrigerator for relief, you will find that peace in Him.

Let me share an example of this with you. My client Christy was struggling with the loss of both of her parents within two years of each other. She had been their caregiver and had lost sight of taking care of herself in the process. Her focus was on being there for them with whatever their needs were regardless of her own. As she was working to gain back focus on herself, she continued to grieve the loss of them in her life. She also beat herself up for not having been able to keep her weight off while she cared for them. She mourned the loss of not only her parents but herself as well. She was not even sure where to begin to regain control over her health and weight. She would get stuck in the past and allow her thoughts about what should have been or what she should have done to keep her from making forward progress.

To begin correcting her thinking and eating, she first had to acknowledge the story she was telling herself about what all had happened. She had to separate fact from drama. She had to take ownership of what she could and could not do about what had happened. When she spoke of getting through the hard times of watching her parents pass away, she spoke of the strength she felt God had provided her. She said that looking back, only by His grace had she been able to care for her parents as she did. Still she struggled with accepting that her weight gain was part of that process. She beat herself up for not being stronger and for not being able to do the things she needed to for her parents and keep herself in check. This frustration with herself was only sidetracking her from what her current goals were. She wanted to be healthy, feel good, and lose the excess weight she was carrying. In order to do that from a place of love and acceptance, though, she needed to take a different look at the story she was telling about her weight gain. She was going to need to apply the same belief in God's strength that had carried her through caring for her parents to her current situation. She had to recognize that while she could not go back and change the past, she could look at everything that happened from a place of love and belief in God's sovereign plan (Rom. 8:28–29, Phil. 1:6). She needed to trust that God would provide her with the same strength for her current health goals that He had given her to help in taking care of her parents. For her, Philippians 4:13, "I can do all things through Christ who strengthens me," gave her the confidence she needed to move forward, to better understand the pain she had felt over the last few years, and to take the strength from that time as proof of her ability to be strong in this new season. From this place of strength, she made decisions that aligned with her desires for a healthier her.

This is how the connection between feelings and actions plays such an important role in your goals. When you recognize that your actions are different based on how you are feeling, you can then see how your feelings are directly connected to your outcome. If you are taking actions from a place of unwanted emotion, you end up with results that are also unwanted. For example, eating when you are worried or fearful leads to unwanted weight gain and/or an unhealthy relationship with food. When you address your thinking and align your thoughts with God's promises, your feelings align with the actions that will lead you to your desired goals.

Going back to Christy, when she recognized that her strength came from God, not her circumstances, she then honored her body's hunger cues and no longer used food for emotional needs. She had a different level of awareness when other emotions were at the forefront, and she could stop and acknowledge what she was thinking and how she could look at the situation from a different point of view. She was able to lean on the promise of Christ's strength in all things instead of food.

As you learn to apply God's word to your thinking, ask yourself these questions:

- What is the current situation I am facing (fact only)?
- What is the story that I am telling myself about these facts?

- How does this situation make me feel?
- If I react in response to this feeling, what action would I take?
- What happens as a result of these actions?

Then ask yourself:

- What does God's word say? (What truth has He put in your heart?)
- If I believe His word, how does this promise make me feel?
- What actions do I take from this feeling?
- What happens as a result of *this* action?

This will help you see how the only thing that has to change about a situation to have a different outcome is what you choose to believe. You can choose to believe the story you have created, or you can choose to believe God's promises to you.

~The more we apply God's teaching to our lives, the more it becomes part of us.
-Lysa TerKeurst

Chapter 8: A Lens of Gratitude

Hopefully, by this point you have picked up on the theme of perspective. While we may not have control over all of the circumstances around us, we do have control over how we choose to view them and how we choose to react. One of my personal hacks for perspective change is gratitude and choosing to be thankful in all situations (1 Thes. 5:18). It is a practice that I started a while back, and it has changed everything.

Understanding that the perspective I bring to any situation is not only responsible for how I will feel but also for how I will act has shifted my focus immensely. While at one time my goal may have been to justify, to judge, or to change a situation immediately, now, I can bring my awareness back to my thoughts and mind-set and slowly shift the lens of perspective to gratitude. This ability has been strengthened through the practice of "gratitude journaling."

My journey of looking at things through a lens of gratitude began with journaling at night my gratitude from the day's events and has slowly affected how I view each situation. I have learned that I can think however I choose to think about a situation, looking for, and finding, the blessings on purpose. In the good things and the bad things, God is in control and doing His work. You simply must trust Him.

As Jesus Girls, we know that God works out all things for good in the lives of those who love Him (Rom. 8:28); and yes, while bad things happen, He is not responsible for bringing difficulties into our lives. He does allow them, though. He allows the difficulties in order to help us learn and grow, to develop our character further (Rom. 5:3–4), and to reflect Christ in us (James 1:1–13, 2 Cor. 3:18). When my immediate responses are from my own selfish, one-sided perspective, I am not reflecting Christ much. Self-centered responses are the tendency of our human nature because we internalize whatever is going on for us and make it personal. Reality is that the world just does not revolve around us individually, though.

Knowing that God allows challenges in our lives not only to refine us and help us to grow but also to allow us to learn to lean fully on Him grows us into mature Christians (James 1:2–3). The hard times and what we have learned make us able to walk alongside others who may have similar challenges. I know we all think a world filled without challenges sounds pretty amazing, but really, what would that world look like? Relying on God would not be necessary, no real opportunity for connection with God and others would exist, nor would we be able to receive the full blessings of God that these challenges bring into our lives.

If you do not believe me, take a moment and think of something difficult you went through in the last few years. Imagine that it had never happened. What would your life look like now? Anything and anybody in your current life that was a result of that event would no longer be there. Your life would look nothing like it does right now. In fact, there is no telling what your life would look like without the series of events that happened as a result of that situation.

My struggle with weight and food has enriched my life in more ways than I can even count. Even though this has been a lifelong battle, so much of what makes my life so joyful and full right now is directly connected to that battle. If I had no yo-yoed my way into my thirties, everything from meeting my trainer (and now friend), whom I met when I started my last weight loss journey more than eight years ago, to the fact that I am now a life coach and weight loss coach would have never happened. None of these facts, nor the friends, events, and experiences I have been blessed with since then would have happened. I am not saying that those years were not filled with sadness and difficulties too; but those experiences not only made me a stronger person, they also drew me closer to God in my personal walk and allowed me the privilege of walking alongside other women who have similar struggles.

This journey has not only revealed to me my strength through Christ, but it has clarified to me the purpose for which God put me on this earth: to love, share, connect, and serve those around me. He also desires for me to have compassion for everyone else's struggles because we all have them and to ground myself in God's truth, promises, and love. Had my life been picture-perfect with no problems at all, I am not sure how rewarding it would be. Without the struggles, how are we able to fully enjoy the gift of God's promises? How are we to understand what love really feels like? How would we ever be able to have compassion for others?

Gratitude in *all* things is an opportunity to reframe the purpose of your struggle and to choose a different way. Struggle is defined as "difficulty handling or coping with." When we choose to take God's perspective through His promises, struggle becomes a choice. This does not mean that life will not still bring about difficulties and challenges but that *struggling* with the challenges is a choice. You can choose whether to resist and fight against what is happening or to move forward with not only the knowledge that God is at work in this challenge with you but also the knowledge that you have the power of His strength and the promise of His blessing. You can face any challenge with an understanding that you are equipped with everything you need to face the "struggle" and find the blessings in it.

Keeping a gratitude journal is a great way to start this shift in perspective. Not only does it give you the opportunity to reflect in the morning or evening (or both) on what you have to be grateful for, but it also gives you a chance to start looking for blessings in the struggle and to see the struggle as God at work in your life. Journaling may enable you to lean deeper into Him for understanding and to connect with His purpose in what may be going on in your life. Sometimes staying in the short-term vision of what might be going on is natural; but when you can zoom out and start to look at the bigger picture of what is happening and why, you start to see that God is working a much bigger puzzle than you can see right now.

His vision is infinite (Is. 46:9–10); He is able to see how putting one specific puzzle piece in place changes the whole picture while you are stuck just looking at the one individual piece of the puzzle. The edges, the curves, the holes, with that one piece you are holding, you cannot see how your piece fits into anything at all much less something beautiful. It does, though, and God has already promised you that. You just have to believe Him. Some of the pieces we will get to see in play Often times, we will not on this side of Heaven; but He has promised you good; He has promised you a reward; He has promised you victory. If you choose to trust Him, you can be He is creating a pretty amazing picture.

- Begin a gratitude practice by journaling daily Make a commitment to do this for at least 30 day

and notice the shift in your mind-set.
- Identify what time of day works best for you and commit to writing at least three things that you are grateful for from the day. There is no wrong or right way to do this. The blessings may be written in one word, or you may end up journaling about each blessing. I actually do both. Some days I write a series of words to represent what I am grateful for from the day, and other days I journal about events from a place of gratitude.
- Consider thanking God for things which you have prayed for but have not yet seen answered. Trust that He is working on these blessings.
- Practice looking at every situation through a lens of gratitude.

~Gratitude makes sense of our past, brings peace for today, and creates a vision for tomorrow.
-Melody Beattie

Chapter 9: Be Still and Know

Stillness is not a virtue that our society teaches much, nor does our everyday life normally reflect it. The ability to get still, take a breath, and connect with God's presence is a skill that will take you through all of life's twists and turns with intention, though. Too often we are in reactive mode. Our plans change, stress hits, we get a call we are not expecting, a fight happens with our spouse or family, and we immediately react. We do not even bother to take a breath, to adjust, or to be intentional in our response.

This is the type of situation where the benefits of prayer and meditation step in. In order to benefit from these two things in a crisis, we need to be practicing them in our daily, non-reactive lives. We need to make taking time to sit still with God and our thoughts a daily priority in our lives, another nonnegotiable that we make sacred. There are so many things as a Jesus Girl that we feel like we *need* to do to be right with God. I hope by now you know that loving and accepting Jesus is all that is required, but just because you have the foundation right does not mean that our hearts do not *want* to do more things to be close with God and to experience Him on a daily basis. While your schedule may tell you that you do not have time for such things, the longing on your heart serves a very important purpose to this journey. God is asking you to take time for Him, to get quiet and acknowledge His presence, to turn to Him with the prayers on your heart, and to recognize that He is waiting. He wants you to intentionally choose to turn to Him and discuss whatever is on your heart and mind.

So often we have trained ourselves to distract ourselves, to numb out, or to turn to someone else (spouse, best friend, mom, etc.) when the world has thrown something at us and we want to vent and/or react immediately instead of taking a second to adjust. I know in the moment that not just reacting seems impossible, but this is where we have to not only discipline our actions but also our thoughts. We have to remember that God is in control and has equipped us with everything we need to react in a Spirit-guided way, responding to whatever is going on with love, kindness, and self-control, and to reflect the fruits of the Spirit.

The question remains, then, how do you take a second to breathe? How do you remind yourself in that moment of intense emotion that God has your back? How do you turn directly to Him in that situation instead of lashing out or turning directly to food? Responding correctly requires the strength of a daily practice of prayer and meditating on God's word. The strength is built through setting aside time each day to get quiet and reflect and talk to Him.

Think about the last time you blew up and got frustrated, sad, or anxious. What did you do? Did you cry, eat, pout, or start texting or calling someone to vent? Would you label these reactions as an intentional choice or a habit? Are you happy with these decisions, or do you wish you would have responded differently?

In a perfect world, how would you like to respond when the world throws a curve ball your way? It will, you know. Our best laid plans are still just plans. We all know that things do not always go the way we wish, but how we respond is completely within our control. God has given us the free will to decide how to act, and thinking precedes action.

Unfortunately, we fail to even take a moment to *think* clearly before we take action many times. Especially in the negative times when things throw us off balance and life seems to blow up, we tend to respond out of habit, not with intention.

Your ability to think clearly requires stillness; it requires a moment to process, to acknowledge your thoughts, and to listen to the Holy Spirit's leading. Renewing of your mind is not a "one and done" type of thing. It is a daily commitment to reading God's word, praying for His guidance, and listening for the whispers of the Holy Spirit (Rom. 12:2; Ps. 63:1; Ps 46:10). Even then, you will still have a choice. You can choose to listen to the Holy Spirit or to do things your way. Fortunately, you have a forgiving and patient God (Ps. 78:38–39); and even when we go about doing things our way first, He will be there to correct us and allow us a second (or third) chance (Pr. 24:16a).

So how do you go about making this a daily practice? It is pretty easy actually. It starts with simply talking to God, taking time each and every day (or throughout the day) to stop and pray to Him. The prayers can be prayers of thanksgiving, requests for guidance and wisdom, and even tears of frustration and confusion. He wants to hear it all even though He already knows what you are thinking (I Pt. 5:7). He still wants us to come to Him and trust Him with the good, the bad, and the ugly.

He wants us to be curious, to want to learn, and to grow closer to Him. He is not going to force you into a close relationship; the choice is always yours (Rev. 3:19–20). As you continue to grow that prayerful relationship, you experience Him and all of His promises for you. As you learn and meditate on His word, you feel the peace that He promises, a peace that passes understanding (Phil. 4:6–7). You understand that while you might not know what is going on in a certain situation, you can trust that His plan is good and that He has your back. Spending daily time devoted to building this relationship with Him and learning what His Word says is what will enable you to react differently than you have in the past. You will be able to stop in the moment of anxiety and turn to His promises that you have stored up in your heart (Ps. 119:11).

God created us as intellectual beings. Our minds are exceptional. They have the ability to work not only instinctively but also habitually. Our brains are wired to work as efficiently as possible. The downside to this efficiency is that our brains will help us to build a habit regardless of whether it is healthy for us or not. However, the good news is our brains are flexible in the sense that we can continue to train them to do new things. Dr. Caroline Leaf is both a Christian and a neuroscientist who has worked for years researching how the brain works and its ability to learn new processes. As her research shows, we can truly learn to think and act in new ways. We have the ability to intentionally choose our thoughts, and in doing so we can practice new ways of thinking that are aligned with God's truth.

As a Jesus Girl, you no longer have to carry those limiting thoughts and habits around. You get to choose what new habits you want to form: habits of depending on God instead of food, habits of taking a breath in a time of crisis to reframe what is going on through God's truth, and habits of walking daily with Him in an intimate and personal way. Through these intentional habits you will experience God completely and begin to replace the old patterns with His truth and love.

- Begin to pray to God throughout the day. B

intentional about talking to Him as things come up in your day. Ask for guidance; thank Him for your blessings; call out to Him with all of your needs.
- Set aside time daily, at least ten minutes, for devotional time. With curiosity, begin to read His Word and learn more about His promises to you.
- Ground yourself in His truth, love, and promises daily. Set your intention to react in situations from this place of connection with Him

~The quieter you become the more you can hear.
-Ram Dass

Chapter 10: Mercy and Grace

"Amazing grace, how sweet the sound . . ." Grace is such a beautiful, life changing, soul shaking gift. I think sometimes that wrapping our brains around this unearned blessing is so hard for us that we allow the confusion to stop us from showing ourselves the same love. To understand God's love for us through His gift of grace is mind-blowing and awe-inspiring at the same time. His grace is a blessing that we do not deserve given by the sacrifice of His Son (Eph. 2:8–9). When was the last time you sat with this gift, held it in your arms, and gazed at it with your full attention?

His grace and mercy are really the most unbelievable blessings that any of us can imagine. To have the Creator of the universe care so much about each and every one of us that He knows the details of our lives, and loves and accepts us because of who we are, not in spite of, is just mind-boggling. He meets us exactly where we are with the mercy of forgiveness and compassion and then gives us the ultimate gift of love and eternity with Him through grace (Ps. 145:9). Even if we cannot quite wrap our brains around this truth, the reality is not changed. It *is* true, and it is a gift that is available to us with no questions asked. We do not have to earn the forgiveness and love. We do not have to prove our worthiness for them. We are His—and because we are His, His grace and mercy become ours as part of our inheritance.

Not only does this gift of mercy and grace provide a direct connection to Him, but they are also the perfect examples of the relationship He offers us with ourselves. When we allow His love to transform us from the inside out, we are conduits of this blessing to ourselves and others. We are walking examples of mercy and grace.

Sometimes we struggle with allowing these gifts to be our guiding light, a guidance that allows us to show kindness to ourselves while also being empowered to change and understand that we are still human, that we will falter, and that we will fail at times. Failure does not have to mean anything more than the decision we made did not turn out the way we had hoped or that a different approach might have worked better. Failure is a part of life and learning. It is a requirement for success and growth. To make decisions and learn from them is the best gift we can give ourselves. We also need to be willing to forgive ourselves when we fail.

I wish I could tell you that you will not stumble and that your path will be completely clear from here on out with no detours or pot holes. Unfortunately, chances are very good that you will encounter a few speed bumps and blocks in the road. You will, at times, make a decision with the best of intentions that just does not work out. At times, your past struggles with food and your weight will rear their ugly heads, or plans will change. This does not have to mean failure or struggle. This does not have to mean that anything has gone wrong. In fact, your ability to stay open and prepare for these events to the best of your ability, will allow you to learn the most from them.

When you do find yourself in one of these moments, the perfect opportunity has come to slow down. If the food is in your hands and headed to your mouth, you can always stop and take a break and assess what is really going on. If you find you have already overeaten, take time to reflect, to forgive yourself, and to learn from the experience. What thought were you thinking in that moment? What feelings were driving you to eat? Make those connections and take note for future times. Allow yourself to grow stronger from the situation. This is not turning a blind eye to what is going on. This is intentionally choosing mercy in the moment and allowing God's grace to change you.

If you find yourself upset over what the scale reads or the fact that you are not losing weight as fast as you would like, check in with yourself as to why you are frustrated. What story are you telling yourself about that scale weight? What expectation have you put on yourself (and why) for losing weight? What feeling are you chasing in that moment that does not feel available to you? Remember, your feelings come from your thoughts, not the scale or your weight.

If you get "off track" with making exercise a priority, revisit your reasons for why you want exercise to be a part of your life. What purpose do exercise and movement serve for you? What do you need to believe about moving your body to make it a priority for you?

When you find yourself disconnected from any area of your life—mind, body, or spirit—identify what is going on with you there. Is there a practice that you had put into place (like journaling or meditation) that maybe you have not been consistently doing? These are not necessarily signs that anything has gone wrong, but just that you need to recommit to the things you have identified as being important to your overall health.

Sometimes you will have circumstances outside of your control that throw you off track. Even once you have a good handle on your power to react in tough situations, you may, on occasion, still act in a way that you wish you had not.

At times things may not flow how you had hoped they would. These will be the perfect times to show yourself some mercy, to allow that beautiful gift of love and peace that passes all understanding to light your way, to be your best friend, to be your best supporter, and to lean heavily on the strength of God (2 Cor. 12:9).

This journey will require you to be kind and patient with yourself. You are healing some areas that have never been addressed. You are unraveling years of beliefs that no longer serve you. You are learning new ways to honor and respect your body. You are rekindling a friendship with the Holy Spirit that lives within you. This will sometimes feel like learning to walk again or, maybe, for the very first time. Some parts of this journey will seem easy, and some will seem hard.

You will have moments where you will get distracted by what the next person is doing or a new, shiny diet/exercise plan. Some days food will seem like "no big deal," and other days will be times that you feel like food is all you can think about. These times will help you grow and learn more about yourself and where your mind is in the moment. You will be able to start making connections to how you react in certain situations to the story you have created in that moment. You will have a new level of awareness as to where your focus has shifted.

These moments will be the perfect opportunity to believe not only in God's goodness but to also hold tightly to His love, promises, and truth. In these moments you will have a choice, and your choice will be to believe in the truth of who you are in Christ and God's plans for you, or to believe the lie that held you back in the past. These times will provide opportunities to intentionally get still, quiet, and reflective

Allow yourself the grace to see the truth in the situation and be open to what role you play in it. Be honest with yourself and God, but not judgmental (1 Jn. 1:9).

Holding on to judgement in these situations is just not helpful and typically leads to a spiral of shame, and shame is a dark, lonely hole that does not allow for growth at all. These moments are when you will want to reach out to someone. Have, or find, a trusted friend who has earned the right to hear your story. Someone to whom you can turn to shine the light of His truth on whatever you are experiencing. Shame cannot survive in the light, and if you are having a hard time getting yourself out of that shame spiral or finding someone you can trust with this part of your life, I am here. Walking alongside you on this journey is an honor and a privilege that I do not take lightly.

I fully understand how hard it can feel to heal all of these parts of yourself, but I also know you can do hard things. You already have done hard things, and you have survived them all. This is no different. God has equipped you with everything you need for this journey including those that can help you. We need to surround ourselves with others that understand and are our cheerleaders, people who truly want to see us heal and shine. While I know sharing these struggles with those around us can make us feel very vulnerable, these are the times in which we grow stronger, for in our weakness, His strength is found. (2 Cor. 12:9)

Please, make a promise to yourself to look around and find people for when you need help. Promise to be your own cheerleader, confidant, and friend; to speak to yourself with the love that He has for you; to use your words in a way that builds you up; and to allow the gifts of mercy and grace to flow freely from Him through you. Mercy is a blessing that will help you thrive in the most difficult times. Grace empowers you to change.

~Grace is what saves us and grows us at the very same time.

Chapter 11: My Prayer for You

My prayer for you, sweet friend, is that you will open your heart and mind to learning a new way, to learning how to listen to your body, to making decisions for yourself from a place of honor and respect, and to trusting your ability to find what healthy looks like for you. I pray that you will rid your mind of the thoughts and beliefs that hold you back and keep you from fully stepping into who you were created to be, that you will understand that your feelings come from thoughts, and that you will remember that you are strong enough to feel your feelings and stop numbing and distracting yourself from them.

I pray that your mind, body, and spirit will stay aligned with your Creator, and through this, bring you healing. He loves you immensely and wants that daily connection with you. He wants to be a part of every decision you make in your life, not to control you, but to guide you with love.

I pray for you to remember that you are so much more than a number on the scale and that the size of your jeans does not dictate your worth or how big of a blessing God has for you and can do *through* you. My prayer is that by applying God's promises and truth to your life you will find the feelings for which you long, the feelings you thought would only come from achieving a certain weight goal. My hope is that you will learn to experience joy, love, peace, and purpose as your birthright, not as something you have to earn.

I pray that you understand that you are perfect in His eyes. He wants you to see the image He sees in you, not the image the world may try to reflect back to you. His plans for you are far greater than anything you can imagine, more than your dreams come true. When you lean on Him, He will reveal His plan to you piece by piece. Without distractions, you will be able to experience the true gift of this life He created you for.

I pray that you will be kind to yourself in this process, that you will show yourself the same amount of mercy that has already been given to you through Jesus, that you will look at your life and all the experiences in it through a lens of gratitude, that you will see that every situation has a distinct blessing specifically created for you, that life has no mistakes. Everything happens for a much greater purpose. God is for you, and nothing formed against you will prosper.

I pray that through this journey you will experience true healing; that you will let go of the chains you have carried mentally and physically, chains which have already been broken; and that you will lay your burdens at the cross and leave them there. Remember that you get to define what a healthy mind, body, and spirit look like for you and that this definition can change as the seasons of your life change.

I pray that you will fully embrace the truth that God created you for a purpose. He has a plan for you. He is with you and never will forsake you. You are not alone in this journey. Many other Jesus Girls are walking this path with you, and we are here to light the way for each other, to support each other, to lift each other up when we feel weak, and to remind each other of our purpose and importance.

I pray that you will fully step into the Jesus Girl that you are, fearfully and wonderfully made, clothed with strength and dignity, and created in His image.

And if you have never accepted Christ as your Savior,

pray that you will take this moment to turn to H[im]
His free gift of salvation. The Bible says, "If you c[onfess with]
your mouth, 'Jesus is Lord,' and believe in your hear[t that God]
has raised Him from the dead, you will be saved" (Ro[mans 10:9]).
With an open heart, pray this simple prayer to Him, "De[ar God,]
I call out to you. I'm a sinner in need of a Savior. I repent [of my]
sins and accept your free gift of forgiveness and heaven [one]
day. I accept Jesus into my heart as Lord of my life. Thank y[ou]
for sending your Son to make a way for me to have th[is]
personal relationship with you. I commit my life to you. It's in
Jesus name I pray, Amen."

Welcome to the family, sweet Sister. His healing is for you. He will never leave you. You are a Jesus Girl.

Made in the USA
San Bernardino, CA
03 March 2018